CONFESSIONS
OF A
PARK AVENUE
PLASTIC
SURGEON

CONFESSIONS OF A PARK AVENUE PLASTIC SURGEON

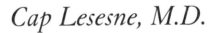

Cap Lesesne, M.D.

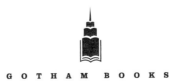

GOTHAM BOOKS

GOTHAM BOOKS
Published by Penguin Group (USA) Inc.
375 Hudson Street, New York, New York 10014, U.S.A.
Penguin Group (Canada), 90 Eglinton Avenue East, Suite 700, Toronto, Ontario, M4P 2Y3 Canada
(a division of Pearson Penguin Canada Inc.); Penguin Books Ltd, 80 Strand, London WC2R 0RL, England;
Penguin Ireland, 25 St. Stephen's Green, Dublin 2, Ireland (a division of Penguin Books Ltd.);
Penguin Group (Australia), 250 Camberwell Road, Camberwell, Victoria 3124, Australia (a division of Pearson
Australia Group Pty. Ltd.); Penguin Books India Pvt. Ltd., 11 Community Centre, Panchsheel Park,
New Delhi—110 017, India; Penguin Group (NZ), cnr Airborne and Rosedale Roads, Albany, Auckland 1310,
New Zealand (a division of Pearson New Zealand Ltd.); Penguin Books (South Africa) (Pty.) Ltd.,
24 Sturdee Avenue, Rosebank, Johannesburg 2196, South Africa

Penguin Books Ltd., Registered Offices: 80 Strand, London WC2R 0RL, England

Published by Gotham Books, a division of Penguin Group (USA) Inc.

First printing, October 2005
10 9 8 7 6 5 4 3 2 1

Copyright © 2005 by Cap Lesesne, M.D.
All rights reserved

LIBRARY OF CONGRESS CATALOGING-IN-PUBLICATION DATA
has been applied for.

ISBN 1-592-40170-8

Printed in the United States of America
Set in Granjon
Designed by BTDNYC

PUBLISHER'S NOTE
All names and identifying characteristics have been changed to protect the privacy of the patients involved.

This book is dedicated to

JOHN M. LESESNE, M.D.,

and

DAVID C. SABISTON, M.D.,

physicians worthy of emulation

I believe in strict patient confidentiality. To honor this principle, names and circumstances have been altered, and the identities of patients are known only to me. In those cases where patients have permitted their names to be used, I have done so.

The names of institutions, teachers, colleagues, staff, and friends are real. The same is true for celebrities—except, again, where they have also been patients.

Contents

Acknowledgments

▼ ▼ ▼

I gratefully acknowledge the invaluable assistance of the staff at Gotham Books—in particular, Bill Shinker, Lauren Marino, and Hilary Terrell—without whose encouragement and help this book would never have happened. I am similarly grateful to Matthew Guma of Inkwell Management for his skill and enthusiasm.

I am deeply indebted to the many professors and mentors I've been fortunate enough to encounter through the years.

I could not do what I do without an exceptional staff. I wish to thank all those who've assisted me in the past, and who so expertly continue to do so today.

Above all, I'm indebted to my patients. They are not merely foremost in my mind. They have made my life worthwhile.

Preface: On the Table

▼ ▼ ▼

The nightmare every surgeon dreads is coming true, before my eyes. My patient is dying.

And I don't know why.

Lee McKenzie, a seventy-year-old Manhattanite and former literary agent, lies sedated on the table in my operating room. Maybe she's dreaming about the face-lift she's undergoing, and for which she's saved up over many years. She couldn't have been more certain that the operation would recharge her. She'd said so months before, when she'd visited my office at the urging of a friend on whom I'd done an eyelid lift. "Feeling ugly and rejected is no way to go through life," said Lee. I wouldn't have been shocked had she dumped a lifetime of accumulated coins and bills on my desk right there.

Lee had an unusually heavy neck, baggy eyelids, and lots of jowl, and very much looked her age. Observing her both in person and in photographs at age forty and forty-five, I determined we'd get the best outcome—a defined neck, with chin and jawline clearly separate from the neck—by removing fat from the platysma muscle between her clavicle and jaw, pulling the largely functionless muscle backward, and removing extra fat along the jawline. It's an operation I've performed maybe three thousand times. Barring complications, she would be off the table and in the recovery room within three and a half hours from the moment she was wheeled into my OR. Bruising and swelling would be gone within two weeks, and she would look as if she'd bought seven to ten years.

Before I could operate, though, we had to confirm she was up to it. Her health, generally, was excellent. She had never smoked.

Never had a heart problem. The preoperative tests—EKG, blood studies, stress test—all turned up normal. The morning of the operation, she was so excited she practically wheeled herself into the OR.

Now, a couple hours later, I am also experiencing a rush, but it's because Lee is lying on my table just beneath me, her face opened from ear to mouth, and something is going very wrong.

The operation is still an hour from completion. I have finished removing fat and elevating the skin on her right side, and I am doing the same on the left when Lisa, my trusted anesthesiologist of fourteen years, says, "I have a problem."

"What is it?" I ask.

"Her blood pressure's dropping, her oxygen's dropping, and I can't reverse it."

"What do you mean you can't reverse it?"

"I've reduced the anesthetic, I've increased her fluid, I've given her medicine to bring the BP up, and it won't go above ninety over fifty."

"Let's put her on one hundred percent oxygen," I say.

Lisa does—to no avail. Two minutes later, Lee's O$_2$ level is still low and her blood pressure is down to 80/50.

My hands are moving as fast as possible. It's not abnormal for patients to have brief episodes of low oxygen or blood pressure, but this one is persisting. I can't simply stop operating. I have to close her up. And before I can do that, I have to stop the bleeding.

"I'm getting worried," Lisa says. "Hurry up." Like most anesthesiologists, Lisa is paid to be, among other things, cool. We've been through a lot and we trust each other; I've done face-lifts and other procedures on friends she's referred to me. But the mix of symptoms manifesting in Lee is new to both of us. My mind runs through the possible explanations.

Heart attack? Maybe, but her EKG hasn't changed.

Aspiration? Doesn't jibe with the drop in BP.

Vasovagal syncope? Her O$_2$ would be normal.

Could this be Lee's normal blood pressure? Still doesn't explain the oxygen drop.

Something going on in her head or nervous system? She has no history of neurological problems.

Pulmonary embolism? She's too physically active for a blood clot. Even though Lee's EKG hasn't changed, I go with the most reasonable possibility: heart attack. After twenty-plus years in training and private practice, this is, remarkably, the first time a patient of mine is suffering a heart attack midsurgery.

"Reverse all the anesthetic," I tell Lisa. She shuts down the standard cocktail of fentanyl, propofol, and Versed that had ushered Lee into a "twilight" sleep, while I speedily continue closing incisions, tying fine nylon sutures, and inserting nickel clips in the scalp. Finally, Lee's blood pressure begins to rise. Same with her O$_2$. Good. The sedation has worn off and it's only local now. As Lee awakens—the still-opened side of her face resembling a cut watermelon—she asks groggily, "Are we done?"

"We have a little problem," I say.

"What problem?"

"Do you have chest pains?"

"No."

Huh. Another indicator she did not have a heart attack.

"Shortness of breath?" I ask.

"No. What problem?"

"We didn't like some of the readings," I say.

Lee looks at me as if I were dense, as if I were from Neptune— as if I've forgotten why we are all gathered there and why I have gone into this profession to begin with. As if I've forgotten why she has spent every last discretionary penny to be lying here.

"I don't care if I die," she says. "I waited my whole life to look good. I'm not going one more day looking the way I do."

Her eyes are piercing; there are no remnants of the effects of anesthesia. "Just do a good job," she coaches me.

Despite her aberrant readings, I accede to Lee's wish and complete the face-lift. This time, her signs remain stable. After I finish and suture her, we call for an ambulance to transfer her to the hospital, to make sure she's monitored.

The moment the EMS technicians place Lee on a stretcher—the face-lift dressing cradling her head—her eyes roll back and she turns blue.

Oh, God, I think. *She's gonna go.*

She *is* having a heart attack.

Fortunately, Lee responded to another drug-reversing agent. She came to; she did not code. That night, in a crowded emergency room, with an IV in her arm, she asked me, "Did you do a good job?" It's a question she would ask me every day for the week it took her to recover in the hospital's cardiac care unit.

I nodded.

"Then I'm happy," she said. "And if I'm not happy, nothing else matters."

CONFESSIONS
OF A
PARK AVENUE
PLASTIC
SURGEON

Introduction

▼ ▼ ▼

We plastic surgeons are perhaps second only to psychiatrists when it comes to being privy to patients' intimate secrets. As a doctor, though, I'm committed to strict confidentiality. Divulging anything is not just unethical, it's illegal: I could lose my license. Indeed, a proper plastic surgeon doesn't even acknowledge his patients when he sees them at events, unless they've been explicitly open about their operation. At a Los Angeles charity function crammed with A-list actors and industry players, several patients of mine roamed the mansion's grounds while I strolled with one of the town's most powerful female executives.

"You're lethal to walk around this party with," she said, taking me by the arm. "I'd love you to comment on who here has done what."

"I can't do that," I said.

She looked at me sternly, as if that might do the trick.

"I can't," I said.

Now she practically batted her eyelashes.

"I can't," I said.*

---

* I can't—though I can tell you a few ways to tell if someone's had plastic surgery:

1. Unevenly dimpled legs. (Liposuction)
2. Symmetrical scars. (Under the armpits: a subpectoral breast augmentation; in the same position on the hips, backs of legs, or fronts of legs: lipo)
3. Scars just in front of the ears. (Face-lift)
4. A break in the hairline. (Face-lift)
5. Facial skin different from skin on top of the hand or, more accurate (since lasers easily remove hand wrinkles and brown spots), different from skin on the lower leg. (Face-lift)
6. Cheekbones too sculpted for overall anatomy. (Cheek implants)
7. Incisions on the tops of the eyelids, sometimes only visible with the eyes closed. (Eyelid lift)

So why would a doctor like me write an exposé about what goes on behind the scenes in my profession?

The last decade, especially the last three to five years, has witnessed a revolution in my profession and its public perception. There's less stigma now to having cosmetic surgery. There are more public expressions of pride by patients. Once upon a time, the only celebrities who confessed to going under the knife were Joan Rivers and Phyllis Diller. It's long been rumored in our circles that the legendary L.A.-based plastic surgeon Dr. Frank Ashley did face-lifts on John Wayne and Gary Cooper (among other Hollywood legends). There was Ann-Margret's obvious facial reconstructive work following her terrible fall in 1972, while rehearsing for a show in Las Vegas. Aside from that, though, there was mostly silence about who'd had work done—and the silence wasn't only from famous folks whose appearance was critical to their livelihood, but the not so famous, too. The high schooler who returned in the fall for her senior year with a suddenly smaller, usually upturned, nose—likely an idealized Caucasian variation modeled on Grace Kelly or Barbie—did not necessarily explain, much less advertise, how the change had come about.

Today, much has changed. Far more people talk openly about the procedures they've had (though many still won't, and some, like Sharon Stone, who sued a plastic surgeon for implying that she might have had work, shudder at the very suggestion). My patients rarely feel the need to disappear for weeks, so they can return to their hometown looking refreshed. In 2004, according to the American Society of Plastic Surgeons, 9.2 million cosmetic surgery procedures were performed in this country, a 24 percent jump from the year 2000. Comparing 2003 to just one year before, almost all major cosmetic surgeries increased markedly: Lip augmentation was up 21 percent; tummy tucks, 18 percent; liposuction, 13 percent; face-lifts, 9 percent; breast augmentation, 7 percent; eyelid lifts, 7 percent. And because of recent technical and medical developments, which have led to the popularity of nonsurgical, outpatient procedures such as "injectables" (in 2003, such minimally invasive procedures jumped 43 percent over the previous year), the decreased cost of beautifying and enlivening one's looks, particularly the face, is increasingly attracting the nonwealthy. Those who might once have chosen a forehead lift (average national fee: $2,800) are opting instead to get a Botox injection ($375 every five months).*

Yet despite the more accepting attitude toward cosmetic surgery, and despite the booming business my profession is enjoying, the surgeon—the good one, anyway—remains behind the scenes. For most patients, the goal is subtlety, and the doctor who delivers subtle results is greatly appreciated—discreetly.

To repeat, then: Why would a doctor like me write an exposé?

Because of my experience as a plastic surgeon and my particular skill—to reposition the skin and tissue of the face, to sculpt fat, to reverse the residuals of pregnancy, and to undo some of the other changes wrought by time—I have come to see, hear, and understand an extraordinary amount about the range of our dreams and disappointments, our motivations and fears. Two decades of solo plastic surgical practice have exposed me to the yearnings of the human heart. While I'm a technician who transforms his patients physically, I also bear witness to their psychological transformation, which frequently starts before the bruising has resolved. For instance, a woman having breast augmentation often sees such a radical upswing in confidence and body image, she makes another dramatic change: new boyfriend, new job. Why? Often, her man becomes more interested in her—*way* more. Indeed, a husband

---

* In the long run, the forehead lift is probably cheaper.

may become so infatuated with his wife's new breasts that she may perceive his lust as weakness. She may lose respect for him. I can't count how many times I've seen it happen.

On the other hand, couples that come in together for cosmetic surgery—a small but not insignificant part of my practice—almost always display some of the healthiest relationships and long-term intimacy I've ever encountered.

Like it or not, I'm exposed to my patients' lives before, during, and after surgery. You know many of them from magazine covers, movies, and TV. Some of them walk the fashion runway. Some run for office. Some are royalty. Some are rock stars. Some are socialites. Some are international tycoons. You've seen their boldfaced names, or those of their spouses, in the gossip columns and the business pages. My practice is located in the epicenter of the plastic surgery world—an eight-block stretch along Park Avenue between Sixty-fourth and Seventy-second streets where the major players have discreet offices that cater to (among others) the wealthy, the famous, and the beautiful.

And the often unhappy.

I am not a psychiatrist, nor do I have Oprah's gift for empathy. I am not overly warm and fuzzy—an occupational necessity rather than a character flaw. But I have sat and listened and tried my best not to judge as prospective patients have come into my office and shared with me their aspirations, the physical attributes that haunt them, and other insecurities. They tell me their stories, proving that even the most successful, attractive, and seemingly aloof people suffer many of the problems that haunt all of us, regardless of status. We all share the identical fears about appearance, age, and time. We worry that our looks or aging will lose us love, security, desire, or sexual attractiveness. He can't get the movie role he wants. She can't get a date. He's been working out for six months and still has an abdominal roll. She comes to me after a divorce or on the eve of menopause. He comes to me not long before he's up for a promotion, or right after he doesn't get it. She's about to cheat on her husband, though he doesn't know it; in fact, *she* doesn't yet know it. (What else am I to make of a comely young woman, half-French, half-English, who repeatedly complains to me about her investment banker husband, and who describes her intensive spinning class and free-weights regimen—her first serious exercise since giving birth five years before—and yet insists that the face and breast surgery she desires are "only for herself"?)*

Many of my patients are between forty and sixty, with the rest divided evenly between those older and younger. Women are particularly vulnerable during these decades. Their childbearing years are nearly over. Their kids are getting older. Their parents may be dying. They've become the elders, the generation in charge. Patients sit in my consult room and tell me things not even their husbands or girlfriends or best friends know. Essentially, they want me to restore a lost youth, back to when they were nineteen, or twenty-six, or thirty-five, or forty-seven. Their determination to rediscover happiness and self-assurance supersedes all else. "If I don't look good after this face-lift," said Lee, the seventy-year-old who shrugged off the *heart attack* she'd had immediately following her operation, "then nothing matters."

I maintain a familiarity with my patients for brief periods or for much longer. Frequently, I get to know them well—maybe too well. I become friendly with many, travel with them, attend their weddings and even those of their children. Sometimes I'm invited to their postdivorce parties. It's no wonder such a bond should form between patient and doctor. In doing something so intense and personal, and which can palpably improve lives, I can't help but achieve

---

* Six months later I spot her at The Ivy in Los Angeles. She's having a romantic dinner with a younger man.

a closeness unusual for doctor and patient. For my patients' part, they can't help but reveal themselves candidly to me. Part of this intimacy stems from the fundamental difference between elective and nonelective surgery. By the time prospective patients have chosen to appear in my office, they've thought deeply about personal and often painful subjects—their self-perception, how others regard them, and their goals.

During our introductory consultation, the patient and I will share pleasantries, then she'll switch gears. For example, Renee, forty-two, suddenly tells me, "I'm meeting my old high school boyfriend next week, and I don't look as good as I want to. Can you do a liposuction of my abdomen and legs and fat grafts for my lips in time?" (I can.) Or Frank, a New York TV anchorman, orders me to make him look younger by removing the fat bags in his lower eyelids, after his production manager comments on Frank's late-night carousing—a particularly deflating comment since Frank spends his nights at home, prepping for work. (On-air TV personalities require a different surgical and aesthetic approach—more on that later—so I remove the fat by making incisions inside the eyelids. After surgery, Frank looks five years younger, with no visible scars, and misses only one weekend of work.) Or Danielle, a once beautiful, newly widowed social force in Palm Beach, complains that because of a disastrous surgery performed on her by a non-board-certified plastic surgeon, her face has deteriorated into a distorted, unnatural mask, with sweeping lines across her cheeks. "I'm desperate," she says. "You have to help me." (When I cut the multiple suspension sutures that distort her smile, her cheeks release and resume a more natural position; the results are apparent before the surgery is even done.)

And then there's Liz.

A five-foot-five, seventy-three-year-old dynamo and legend in the public relations field, Liz seemed particularly pleased with my operations. She had asked me to change her breast implants three times in two years and was always happy with the way they turned out. A little smaller, a little bigger, then smaller again. C cup, now C+, now down to a B+. Although I initially balked at the second and third surgeries, Liz's motivation seemed appropriate, and after much discussion, I believed she understood the limitations and risks (e.g., asymmetry, hardening, infection, bleeding) of each surgery.

Still, Liz looked somewhat anachronistic: youthful breasts on an aged body. But while this might tweak my aesthetic sense, Liz didn't see it that way. She was thrilled.

I was neither flattered nor dismayed by Liz's desire to routinely change her breast implants, but I was curious. I continued to probe for the reason behind the frequent adjustments. For more than two years, I got no satisfactory answer from her.

Six months after the third surgery, Liz comes to the office to discuss new implant set number four—and finally she cops to her motivation. "I change my breast size depending on who I'm dating," she admits.

"Liz, I can't do this anymore," I tell her.

"Why do you care? It doesn't hurt me, and it makes me feel good. Please," she begs. "Just one more time."

"No. Three is enough." Each time an implant goes in, the body forms a layer, or capsule, of collagen, which can contract and distort the implant. While medically and technically there's no reason I can't continue to alter her breast size, I refuse, given her motivation, to do more surgery.

Liz scowls at me, not at all thrilled with my admonition.

"Can't you put in a zipper?" she wonders.

Just because I want to help my patients doesn't mean I always agree with their "reality." Every now and then, I'm confronted by someone who seems to be looking in a fun-house mirror. Recently, I received this letter from Sapporo, Japan:

> *Dear Dr. Lesesne,*
> *I understand you are a famous plastic surgeon.*
> *My daughter looks like Elizabeth Taylor.*
> *I would like her to look more Japanese.*
> *Can you make her look more Japanese?*
> *Thank you.*
> *Sincerely,*

It was signed by the girl's mother.

Stapled to the letter was a photograph of a homely, very Japanese-looking fourteen-year-old girl.

Thanks to my unusual access to people seeking significant physical changes, I write this book, in part, to share what I've learned about what motivates us and what terrifies us.

My subjects are women and men seeking plastic surgery; my subject is the skin and tissue of aging faces and bodies. Over the course of my years in practice, I've seen an almost incessant burst of innovation—including lasers, Botox, collagen, Sculptra, Restylane, short-scar surgery, and endoscopic surgery—that has helped to improve results dramatically, while reducing bruising, scarring, and recovery time. Other medical innovations not specifically intended for plastic surgery have also helped the quality of the work and the patient experience. For example, the pulse oximeter, a device that measures the blood's O_2 level, allows us to monitor anesthesia continuously, thus making for safer, more accurate administration of sedation, as well as allowing for more office-based surgery. Versed, a Valium derivative, and fentanyl, a narcotic, have gained popularity because they are short-acting; when the surgery is over and we cease sedation, the aftereffects for the patient are gone within an hour, not days.

But it's not just technical innovations and new drugs and the latest injectables that tantalize my patients. I've come to understand, after thousands of operations, a great deal about the anatomy of the face that isn't found in anatomy textbooks. I've learned about light and shadow. About the way skin heals. About skin tension. About how much fat to remove (and whether to excise it or suction it). About where and why a surgeon should leave extra skin. About how best to disguise scars. About the false expectations of computer imaging. About why it's crucial to examine the face over time and not just in the present. About which skin regimens work and which don't. About a myriad of other lessons, large and small. All that knowledge has made my surgery of the face, in particular, far better today than when I did my first face-lift, in the winter of 1980, as a new surgical resident at Stanford University, assisting on a standard subcutaneous lift of a fifty-two-year-old mother of three.

I also believe that there are strategies, in contrast to those of some of my colleagues, that allow me to achieve more natural results. "Where did Greta Van Susteren go?" patients of mine wondered, along with many others, even after the Fox TV anchor admitted to eyelid procedures (she never confessed to more). "Please don't make my mouth like Melanie Griffith's," patients will demand before I inject their lips with Restylane. Or they might ask me, "What happened to Meg Ryan?" (Angelina Jolie's name is also invoked, but in her case it appears the lips are her own.) The obviously plasticized look is not the usual goal of my patients; subtlety makes them happy. "Natural" is my guiding aesthetic principle. For facial surgery, my goal is twofold: to make my patient look phenomenal, and to make no one suspect why she looks phenomenal. I want her to be able to pull her hair back without any visible scars. A patient from Texas once paid me one of my favorite compliments: "You made me look younger, intellectual, *and* sexy."

On the other hand, I find it comical that so many women come in for breast augmentation thinking their husband or boyfriend won't know. They're shocked—"Can you believe it?" they ask me—when their partner deduces it in three nanoseconds.

Many surgeons plan their procedures as a matter of routine, without accommodating the patient's physiognomy or individual traits. My profession is degraded, I feel, by practitioners who perform the same style of operation regardless of the subject's nose, face, or body habitus. But there are overbooked surgeons in Los Angeles, Miami, and elsewhere who insert the nearly identical pair of oversize breast implants on a vast cross section of their patients (including office staff, wives, and even daughters), so that every woman who leaves the office sports two half-grapefruits. The result is so artificial that many of us can't help but wonder, "What was the surgeon thinking? What was the *patient* thinking?" Even though I spend all my day with women, and many of my closest friends are women, there are some questions I can't answer.

Then again, other questions that people *think* they have answered, I would challenge. For instance, I believe it's a myth that Michael Jackson is a plastic surgery victim. People assume that everyone believes he's a victim, including Mr. Jackson himself. That he must hate his face (and himself) or else why would he have gone back for more and more and more. . . . You know what I think? That he likes his surgery. A lot. If he'd been unhappy with what was happening to his face and wanted to reverse it, he could have, to an extent. But he never did. He had an idea of what he wanted, and he's been following that road since. We may think it looks bad. I don't believe he thinks so.

Here's another myth: People who have plastic surgery have

complicated feelings about it. No, they don't—not usually. Those who haven't had plastic surgery hyperanalyze the motivations of those who have. For most of my patients, it's a simple decision. They want to fix something that bothers them. Period. No Freudian analysis, no overthinking. Almost every magazine article critical of plastic surgery is usually written by someone who's never felt that urge.

Another reason I write this book is because I've thought deeply about the face, skin, aging, and plastic surgery, and I want to share what I know to be true and false with my patients, with those interested in plastic surgery, and with other physicians. Better education about my profession is good for me, my colleagues, and, most important, future patients. Without knowledge, how does a first-time consult know what to look for in a plastic surgeon? Or what to ask the surgeon? I'll include some guidelines.

I love being a plastic surgeon. I love its intellectual demand and technical artistry. Most of all, I love that I make people happy. I'm with my patients every step of the process, for every suture. Many Park Avenue plastic surgeons don't see their patients postoperatively: The resident or post-op nurse treats them. Not me. My mentor at Duke Medical School, Dr. David Sabiston, impressed upon me that they're *my* patients from the moment they enter the OR until the incisions have matured, sometimes more than a year later. As the captain of the ship, I am responsible for anything that happens to them, plastic-surgery-related, while in my care. This simple lesson in accountability has made me a better surgeon because I see changes in healing and other nuances that, were I *not* doing my own follow-up, I might not notice or fully understand. (Two examples: With a smoker who's had a tummy tuck, I can tell sooner, by the shade of blue on her skin, whether she'll have problems with her wound healing. With a face-lift patient, I can tell whether scars need to be massaged.) And because my patients always see *me*, not an unknown, the relationship is more gratifying.

Which brings me to the last reason I write this book: to share what it's like to live the life of a plastic surgeon. Americans have seen slices of it (pun intended) on hit TV series such as *Nip/Tuck*, a fictional drama, and *Extreme Makeover* and *The Swan*. But these programs, both fictional and "reality," offer stylized, often sensationalized, depictions of that life. Among books on the subject, none of those written by plastic surgeons talk in detail about the life we live, its daily rigors and quirks. And books about plastic surgery by journalists, while occasionally well researched, don't come close to capturing the essence of our sense of responsibility to each patient, the numerous details we must consider with each procedure, why we make the decisions we do, and why we make the mistakes we sometimes do. I'll provide an insider's view that outsiders can't, because they don't live it.

For example, how about this paradox to our life: Can one succeed in a profession suffused with one kind of intimacy without also sacrificing—or at least challenging—intimacy in one's personal life? I'm usually scrubbed for surgery before the sun rises, so I have to be in bed early. The society cocktail parties, museum benefits, and charity functions to which I'm often invited—and where I regularly see former and future patients—are, for me, restricted functions. I'm expected to be a diplomat, to be cool and calm, always restrained. It's one glass of wine, tops, and nothing after nine thirty; I'm a doctor. I have to be responsible. I must focus on my surgery.

Even my avocations can be colored by the fact that, like most plastic surgeons, I'm always "on." When I'm at the Metropolitan Museum of Art or the Frick Museum, I wander the halls looking at spectacular paintings and sculpture, yet I can't help but analyze them as if they were patients. The young wife in Peter Paul Rubens' *Rubens, His Wife Helena Fourment, and Their Son Peter Paul* looks overweight; she could use a neck liposuction. Venus in Titian's *Venus and Adonis* is often regaled as the paragon of female perfection, but, to my eye, she's disproportionate. And whenever I see John Singer Sargent's magnificent *Madame X*, which depicts a side view of her large nose with its dorsal hump and flared nostrils, I can't help but think, *What would she look like if I reduced her tip projection and rasped her dorsum?*

This out-of-office PSR—Plastic Surgeon's Radar—is not just operative while I'm strolling the halls of a museum; it's frequently on during social functions, including when I'm having dinner with a woman. It's not long before the more daring of my dates will ask me to comment on what she may or may not need—and sometimes they don't like the reply. One woman, while dancing with me on our second date, challenged me to assess her breasts: "Cap"—my nickname—"what size do you think they are?"

What do I say?

That I know they're 325 ccs? That the implant casings are "smooth" (as opposed to "textured," whose surface features tiny ridges)? That they're of "moderate profile" (the distance of the implants from the chest wall)? That I can even name the implant manufacturer?

"The perfect size," I replied. "They suit you well."

I operate on men and women. I physically and psychologically change them, yet I must remain distant. I champion their initiative and sometimes courage to transform themselves, yet I must be keenly aware of, and candid about, their weaknesses and occasionally misplaced motivations.

My professional obsession is flaws. My goal is perfection.

▼

I agree with Aristotle: The pursuit of life is happiness. Figure out what's important in life, then go for it. If there's a physical attribute that can be fixed, and the procedure involves minimal risk, and your life will be improved because of the fix, then why not do it? I don't trivialize the risk of surgery because all surgery entails risk. But I see, every week, how plastic surgery delivers physical results that change people's lives in positive ways. I love Billy Crystal's famous Fernando Lamas impression on *Saturday Night Live*—"It's better to look good than to feel good." It's funny, at first, because it's about vanity and superficiality. But for many people it isn't far from the truth. For them, feeling good *is* looking good. Attractive physical appearance reinforces good body image, and good body image affects psyche. Others see you in a different light. You may be noticed and appreciated more. You're more likely to get promoted. You get more out of life.

As one face-lift patient told me on a postoperative visit, "This changed my *head*."

Youth (Without Surgery)

▼ ▼ ▼

You aren't born to be a surgeon. There's no natural talent for it. No one is born with a great pair of hands for surgery—for football and piano, maybe; for surgery, no. Usually you become a surgeon (or a doctor, generally) because you want to help people, or because the aspects of the discipline—intellectual, technical, aesthetic, psychological—appeal to you, or because you're lucky enough to have a role model. For me, all three conditions held, though early on, I was aware of only the last of these. My father, John Lesesne (luh-SAYN), was a doctor (now retired), an old-school internist who made house calls in the upper-middle-class suburbs of Detroit, where I grew up in the late sixties, the eldest of six kids. His was the kind of practice, almost obsolete now, where he treated and cared for two, often three, generations of the same family. He was an allergist, specializing in asthma. Sometimes I would go on house calls with him. While Dad paid his visit, I sat in the car, curbside, scanning the windows of the home to see if I could spot him and maybe get a glimpse of what was going on inside, but it was not out of fascination with medicine; it was the fascination of a son for what his father does, a child intrigued by the grown-up world. That's it. At least that's what I thought at the time. Now and then I'd bike by his office and poke in for a visit or, when I got older, stop by St. John's Hospital on Mack Avenue. I had no idea these latter visits would benefit me years later: Because I associated hospitals with Dad's presence, they always felt like places of warmth, even invitation, sanctuaries where people went to get well. For me, a hospital was never the dark, institutional warren of hallways and machines that terrifies most people. It was Dr. John

Lesesne facing a wheezing little boy sitting on a table. "Now take a slow, deep breath through the mouth," my father would urge in his Charleston accent, soft and calm, then place the cup of his stethoscope to the boy's chest.

Proud as I was of Dad, though, as highly regarded as he was in the community, there's another enduring image I have of him, equally unshakable.

It's of him not there.

Because he was always working. Frequently he came home too late for dinner. He would do anything for his patients. He made a good living. I could not respect a man more. But he was anchored in one place, Grosse Pointe, Michigan, a bucolic Midwestern suburb of Detroit, and he would be there for life.

As a kid, I dreamed privately that I was destined for more exotic things.

Throughout my childhood, everyone around me, particularly my friends, seemed to be athletic. I was a klutz at every sport I tried. Rotten at basketball, awful at football and baseball; my hand-eye coordination for sports was terrible. (If someone then had made a bet that my hands would one day be insured against career-threatening injury, so that if anything befell them, I would get $18,000 a month for the rest of my life, he would have made a fortune.) I was the kid to beat up, though mostly I was clever enough to evade pummelings. My outlet was books—about history, foreign affairs, any culture different from mine. I had other diversions—quiet pursuits such as building models and sculpting with clay, those things that boys do if they're not athletes—but mostly it was books. I read constantly. Thanks to these dramas about other places and times, I could dream vividly about the world beyond, and my desire to do something larger-than-life. My grandfather ran a trucking company, and I remember driving around with him through small towns scattered across the Midwest. We would travel to depots where his car-carrying trucks picked up automobiles from the General Motors plants in Flint and Pontiac, then delivered them to car dealers all over the eastern United States. I also remember Teamsters, smashed cars, and Grandpa, baseball bat in hand, once storming out of his car and threatening to kill anyone who would even *think* about intimidating his grandson.

That was exciting.

For a while I thought about going into the family trucking business. But I wanted something removed from Detroit. I was fairly certain my future would have the word *international* attached to it.

In ninth grade, a school friend disappeared—gone, suddenly, to high school far from Grosse Pointe. A prep school in the mysterious East. While it offered a better education than where I was, its more seductive pull was its location: far away. It was just the adventure I ached for. I asked my parents about it. Dad had gone to public schools in South Carolina, Mom to an all-girls private school in Michigan. My father, in particular, was taken by his firstborn's excitement about education and he issued me a challenge. "Work hard," he said, "and I'll pay for the best school you can get into."

Hard work didn't daunt me: I was a diligent student, pulled good grades, woke up early and had jobs on the side—shoveling snow, cutting grass, hauling trash, scooping ice cream. I was fourteen and hungry, and now my hunger for the thrill of a new educational experience had a name to it: Andover.

My first year away was brutal. Overwhelming, lonely, full of awkwardness. It was hard being far from home, at an all-male school, tough living in a dorm, and the courses were difficult. At least I was consistent, though: My first semester there I got a C in everything. I wasn't exactly living up to the bargain I'd struck with my father.

It was hardly any solace to me that getting creamed your first year at Phillips Academy Andover was pretty standard. The campus was gorgeous, pastoral and dreamy in that unsurpassable New England way, with rolling hills and redbrick Georgian buildings, giant shade trees and hockey rinks and a college-caliber library. But at night in the dorms, the school—that first year, anyway—seemed to me a place run by Eastern boys who exacted great pleasure in beating up a bewildered, bespectacled Midwestern outsider whenever they could.

To counter that sometimes helpless feeling, I took up rowing. I knew almost nothing about it. But I'd been curious ever since Dad had told me that his best-conditioned patient was a man named Gus Valenti, who rowed.

At the time, Gus Valenti was eighty-one years old.

Since I was a loser at other sports, rowing made me feel a bit as if Andover was, if not my social haven, then at least an institution where I'd earned inclusion.

As at so many prep schools and Ivy League universities, legacies—offspring of alumni, particularly the well-heeled ones— abounded at Andover. A well-circulated account of an alleged incident during my time there, involving one legacy in particular—from the most powerful family in America—impressed upon me a recurring life lesson: integrity.

No family across the twentieth century has been more associated with Andover than the Bushes, from former president George Bush Sr. through his sons. In my class—class of '73—was Marvin Bush, probably the least well-known of the Bush boys; President George W. (several years ahead of me) and Florida governor Jeb also attended.

In our first year, Marvin (I'd heard) was put on probation for some offense; I believe it was for having a beer in his room. Then, while on probation, Marvin allegedly did yet another thing he wasn't supposed to, thereby violating his probation, which usually meant expulsion. The disciplinary committee convened, and a meeting was attended by students, faculty, administration, and trustees. At the time, George Bush Sr. was head of the Andover board of trustees. Many of the students assumed that, since Marvin's father was head of the board, he'd be cut lots of slack. And, true to form, when the head of the student disciplinary committee stood, he announced that, in the matter of Marvin Bush and his violation of probation, the committee had decided to extend his period of probation. He was spared suspension or expulsion precisely (it seemed to everyone there) because he was a Bush.

Then George Bush Sr. spoke up. "Mr. Chairman," he said, addressing the student head of the disciplinary committee, "if you violate probation, is it customary for your probation to be extended?"

It was a puzzling question since, as head of the trustees—not to mention a former Phillipian himself—he had to know the answer already.

"Well, Mr. Bush . . . no," said the student head of the disciplinary committee almost apologetically.

"I want no preferential treatment for my boy," said Mr. Bush, who then turned to face his son. "Marvin, go back to your room, pack your bag, you're stepping down."

The story raced through the campus. If nothing else, life was getting more exciting.

I rowed. And rowed.

And rowed.

I doubt there's another sport or physical discipline where such a high percentage of participants will volunteer how profoundly it changed their life. I'm one of those. But not because of what happened my first year rowing at Andover. I was awful: the last guy on the eighth and last boat. During my first summer back home from prep school, though, my parents hosted a party, where a patient of Dad's was overheard mentioning that he rowed at the Detroit Boat Club.

Proudly, my father told Mr. Ledyard that I rowed for Andover, conveniently omitting the fact that I was terrible. Intrigued, Mr. Ledyard said that the Boat Club needed an oarsman, and why didn't I come on down to try out for them?

The next morning I met Mr. Ledyard at sunrise. (Only years later did I realize that, as a surgeon who by necessity wakes every day by five, and as a kid who always woke early, the early-bird demands of the sport of crew appealed to my inner clock. I've yet to meet a single successful surgeon or rower who doesn't rise with the sun.) Down at the club, I was assigned to a four-man shell. I was the youngest by seven years.

After an hour and a half, we finished our workout. Mr. Ledyard said they could use me: A boat of theirs had been invited to race in the Canadian Henley Regatta six weeks later and I could fill the slot they were missing.

There was one problem, though. "You're overweight for the boat," said Mr. Ledyard as delicately as possible.

"How much?" I said gamely, not at all offended. I'd never thought of myself as overweight—some baby fat, sure, but I was fifteen and in decent shape, or so I thought. Dropping a couple pounds in a month and a half was no problem, especially for someone who loved his new sport and had grown acclimated to the rigors of crew.

"Forty pounds," said Mr. Ledyard.

Standing on the shore of the Detroit River, sweating after a great workout, excited to be invited to join grown men in an official competition (in another country!)—all in all, I had been feeling like a stud.

But *forty pounds?* The race was on August 5. It was now June 26. Was he crazy?

Although I had one season of rowing behind me, nothing in my life to that point had suggested I was capable of the self-discipline, the torture, I would need to summon to get down to competitive weight. And even if I could find the discipline, was it even physically possible? And if it was physically possible, was it medically smart? I was five feet ten, 185 pounds. The boat, I discovered, was a "lightweight": You *had* to be 145 pounds. If I said I would make weight and didn't, I would fail the boat and the team.

And suppose I did lose the weight . . . how much of my strength would be sapped? They weren't going to want one of their seats manned by a teenager who couldn't pull with maximum strength.

None of these questions mattered. I was possessed.

For the next six weeks, I trained every day, rowing twice a day. I ran. I did weights. I ate almost nothing but vegetables, mostly ones starting with the letter *c.* Celery. Cabbage. Cauliflower. Carrots.

After forty days—weighing in the morning of the race—I tipped the scales at 144.5.

Almost 0 percent body fat. You could count every rib. Forty pounds lighter in forty days.

Barely a third of the way into our race at the Canadian Regatta, in St. Catharines, Ontario, one of the metal clasps that lock the oars in place snapped. Our boat was finished.

All that hard work to finish dead last.

But the experience of earning my way to that seat on that boat on that Canadian lake in August of 1970 imprinted itself on me. Yes, I was a sleeker version of the boy I'd been at summer's start. But the more important development—one that would prepare me for the rigors of becoming a surgeon, perhaps the most competitive of all medical disciplines—was an awakening about obstacles and possibility and fortitude: *If you want it badly enough, you can make it happen.* I'd gotten into a tough prep school by working hard, but this test of will was different. This had involved doing something that *wasn't* pleasurable. This had involved denying myself.

While I may have appreciated, on an abstract level, how this crucible might strengthen me for the future, and perhaps better equip me for professional success later, I certainly did not appreciate how the self-discipline, bordering on ascetic monomania, would implant itself in my life. That is, I may just have succeeded in teaching myself that I could sacrifice so much—perhaps more than I would ever want to, including profoundly important things—to reach my goal.

In the fall I returned to Andover, where the previous spring I'd been the last man on the last boat. I moved up to a stronger boat, and by senior year I was on the first of our "schoolboy eights." We won the New England championship.

As I prepared to go to college at Princeton, I still didn't know what I wanted to be when I grew up. One thing I was sure of, though: being a doctor was not among the options.

At Princeton—leaner and more confident than the last time I'd found myself a neophyte at a leafy, Northeastern bastion of academic excellence—I was ready to test out my new self in a new place.

I studied but still I was lost. My driving priority was to get away from the familiar—perhaps overseas. But I had no idea how I would get there.

I continued to row because I liked it, and because a core self-discipline had been seeded in me as a young teen.

Sophomore year it dawned on me that I had to focus. It was unfair that my parents should pay for four years without something tangible to show for it. After a scattered, generally undistinguished freshman year, I became even more conscious of faraway places. The easiest route to a life of that? I had finally figured it out—and it was right in front of me the whole time:

International law.

With the world-renowned Woodrow Wilson School a mere quarter mile from my dorm, there was no better place to study to be an international lawyer.

This was going to be great, I thought. I would call on my legendary self-discipline from here on in to earn straight A's, work my way to the head of my class, get into a top law school, make law review, win job offers from the most internationally renowned law firms and giant corporations. I'd jet all over the world. I'd live in Paris; all those hours of high school and college French would now come to real use. Someday, when I'd had enough of the bachelor life, I'd marry. We'd live together in Europe and raise a family there.

It seemed like an excellent plan. In the first days back at school sophomore year, I moved into Blair Tower, an all-male dorm and one of the most beautiful, often-photographed buildings on campus. (It's featured prominently in the movie *A Beautiful Mind,* about the brilliant, troubled mathematician John Nash. In fact, during my years there, Mr. Nash would often walk by our door, mumbling to himself.) While some of my dormmates were still enjoying themselves—skiing down six flights of stairs, planning the semester's first road trip to an all-women's college, tossing Frisbees on the quad—I had to tune everything out so that I could be single-mindedly studious. I went to the local lumberyard, bought plywood, and returned to my tiny double. I got out nails and a hammer. I was intent to study, nothing else, for the rest of my college years.

My roommate walked in as I was hammering the first board over my window.

"What the hell are you doing?" he asked.

"Gotta work this year," I said. "See you in nine months."

I boarded over my window except for four inches, at the bottom, for air.

I stopped staying out late on weekends. I even gave up rowing. Too many hours that could be better spent studying.

I still had to eat, though, and I joined one of the college's famous eating clubs—Cap and Gown, which had lots of jocks, male and female. A great deal of social life revolved around mealtime, and I found myself becoming more comfortable in such social settings. Many mornings, for the better part of two years, I ate breakfast with a likable, bright squash player named Meg, who would, in later years, serve as an example to me of the virtue of persistence. I followed news of her, postgraduation, because she married a future surgeon, and we crossed paths on occasion. For Meg, professional success didn't come quite so quickly. She was a businesswoman, but it seemed as if the companies she worked for rarely did very well. She did not let it get her down. Eventually, she was put in charge of a tiny, offbeat company.

It was called eBay.

Meg Whitman is now the CEO of a multibillion-dollar company and one of the most powerful and successful women in the business world.

There were people like that all over campus. To succeed, I was determined to work as hard as anyone.

▼

There was only one little problem concerning my grand plan to become an international lawyer—namely, my prelaw courses.

I despised them. And I was awful at them.

How quickly my dream to be a lawyer crisscrossing the Continent was dashed. Was I abandoning it because it was a new challenge? No. Crew and getting into Princeton and losing forty pounds in forty days proved to me that I didn't shy away from challenges, no matter how tough.

I let go of my "dream" because I would not devote my life to a professional pursuit that I didn't love.

Someday, the dizzying, international life I'd fantasized about would, in fact, become a reality. Meeting an English princess at Ascot. Flying to far-flung parts of the world in private jets to perform work I was trained to perform. Dining with United Nations diplomats and Hollywood directors. Helping one of the most influential and high-profile politicians in America to deal with the one thing he was sure would cost him his career. Accepting a first lady's invitation to cross the country to talk to her. Dating beautiful, intelligent, accomplished women. All of that would be part of my future.

I just didn't know it at the time.

As I finished up my first semester of sophomore year, I was despondent that I truly had no idea of what I wanted to be. And now, suddenly, my boyhood fantasy of mystery and faraway intrigue seemed childish and unsuitable. Little did I know, though, as I took long, broody walks around the Princeton campus, past shade trees and often circling the Institute for Advanced Studies, made famous by Einstein in the fifties, that I was zeroing in on my future. That as I daydreamed while sitting in class, I was mere weeks from discovering my passion. And that that passion, like Dorothy's dream of home in *The Wizard of Oz,* really *was* right there in front of me the whole time.

First Cut

▼ ▼ ▼

After a short lifetime telling myself I was going to do something, *anything,* but be a doctor, which I saw as a dignified, meaningful, admirable, quiet, unadventurous, even boring livelihood, I started to think *only* about life as a doctor. Part of it was the realization, while sitting in science courses in college, that the material came easily and felt so familiar, yet I found it stimulating, too. There were formulas and constants, hard facts and other immutables, but science was always changing, too; one piece of knowledge was always built on the back of another, and another would one day be built on that one. To me, that evolution was more animated and exciting than what I learned in the arts and humanities and social sciences, as much as I enjoyed them.

I had what amounted to another epiphany. Of course, one of the reasons I respected my father and his work so much, and the reason he was respected so much by others, was simple: He helped people. He made their lives better.

My realization? What life could I possibly carve out—crisscrossing the globe, being involved in high-powered deals, you name it—that could outdo, for personal fulfillment, a lifetime of helping people? Dad made kids with asthma breathe a little better, so in the summer they could run around like kids. He helped old people. He helped women and men and families.

I could do that. I wanted to do that.

I'd found something exciting, something important, and something I was passionate about: medicine.

By the time I returned home for Christmas break, my grandmother had got wind of my interest, and she arranged for me to meet Dr. Henry Ransom, a longtime acquaintance of hers who was professor of surgery at the University of Michigan. On a snowy December day, Grandma and I drove the hour and a half through a snowstorm to Ann Arbor, to meet the doctor at University Hospital. Dr. Ransom had grown up on a farm in central Michigan, Grandma told me on the drive, and he was known as a great teacher and an excellent surgeon. He had neither wife nor children. He was in his eighties now, a professor emeritus.

When we pulled into the parking lot, it was the first time I'd ever been to a university hospital, and it was not at all like Dad's hospital—St. John's in Detroit, the inviting, humanly scaled institution my father had been affiliated with since I was a kid, the place I felt so eager to stop in to see him, always feeling comfort inside its walls, even pleasure. But this place, University Hospital, was gigantic, cold, impersonal. For the first time, I understood the anxiety that ripples through most nonmedical people when they set foot inside *any* hospital.

While Grandma and I rode the elevator to the top floor, I wondered if perhaps *this* place wasn't the norm, St. John's the exception, and whether I needed to reevaluate my new, curious, nineteen-year-old's urge to spend the remainder of my waking life in dungeons just like it.

Had you hung a stethoscope around Henry Ransom's neck and slipped a black leather doctor's bag into his hand, you could not have made him look more like the classic physician. When we got to his office, he was sitting behind a big desk, in his white coat. My eyes immediately went to the surgeon's long, thin fingers. Dr. Ransom looked the epitome of an emeritus anything: white-haired, elderly, elegant.

After some pleasantries, the doctor asked about my background. I told him I was at Princeton. Despite my unexpressed reservations in the elevator ride up about the hideousness of University

Hospital as a workplace, I said I'd become interested in pursuing medicine.

"Would you want to work in our department of surgery?" he asked me.

The offer was so sudden, and he knew so little about me, that I thought he deserved an equally impetuous answer.

"Yes," I said, having no idea what the job entailed.

And just like that he was up from behind his desk and motioning for me to follow him. "I want you to meet someone," he said, and we walked into the neighboring office, where a balding, slightly overweight man sat.

"Jerry?" said Dr. Ransom. "I think this young man would be a good researcher."

That was it. My grandmother must have been well regarded by the doctor, I thought, because unless I was wrong, suddenly I had a summer job waiting for me the end of sophomore year, in the department of surgery, at the University of Michigan. And I had yet to take organic chem.

To his credit, the man to whom I'd just been introduced, Jerry Turcotte, the chief of surgery, didn't act put-upon (which said a great deal about his respect for Dr. Ransom). Dr. Turcotte had an easy smile. He'd grown up in Grosse Pointe, too, it turned out, two blocks from my house on Fair Acres Road.

"I know just the spot for you," said Dr. Turcotte. "We're doing research for kidney transplants." Quickly, I was realizing— though I'd had ample evidence to learn it while growing up, from my father the doctor—that medical people, especially surgeons, don't pussyfoot. They don't have time to. They make bold decisions— quick, yes, but bold, first and foremost.

The "research" they had in mind for me that summer, it turned out, did not involve my poring over a bunch of medical texts and data readouts.

They wanted me to cut open dogs.

The doctors in the department were working on an important experiment. They wanted to see if a particular drug, administered just after surgery, would improve the rate of acceptance for kidney-transplant patients. Back then, in the mid-1970s, a kidney transplant was a last-ditch, usually unsuccessful strategy to cure someone suffering from kidney failure. But it was hypothesized that if the patient was given cyclosporine, which reduces the body's rejection of foreign cells, transplants would be much more likely to "keep" and could thus save thousands of lives a year.

Cyclosporine had already been tested on rats, with extremely promising results. It was time to move up the food chain. But before Dr. Turcotte and his team could win approval to test cyclosporine on humans, they would first have to test it on something else.

Dogs. And not just any dog. A specific strain of beagle—one that looked an awful lot like Snoopy from *Peanuts*—was chosen as the, well, guinea pig, because its DNA displayed important similarities to human DNA. Before the dogs were operated on, they were pampered and fed only the best food (should you wonder if the animals were being mistreated). Two surgical teams would work side by side. The dogs were sedated, a pair at a time. Each was spread-eagled, on its back, its paws gently tied back. A breathing tube was placed down its throat. Each surgeon would cut open a dog's abdomen, nudge the intestines aside, and isolate the veins and arteries; this was done by dissecting down to where the artery comes off the aorta and the vein comes off the vena cava—the two main valves leading to and away from the heart. The surgeon would dissect on the ureter (the vessel running between the kidney and the bladder) and cut the blood vessels around the kidneys, to free them. The vessels would be tied and clamped so blood didn't gush out of them. With the kidneys now free, the surgeon would remove them and put them in a bowl, swap bowls with the other team, then plant the foreign kidneys into their new host dog, suture the vessels together, remove the clamps, and make sure there were no leaks (or that we hadn't accidentally sewn a blood vessel to itself). The abdomen would be sewn up. Cyclosporine would be administered.

It was a straight kidney swap. Very science-fictional.

Finally, blood would be drawn from the dogs to see if the new kidneys were working. Was waste being cleared—proof that the kidneys were doing what kidneys should do?

My "research," then, was doing actual surgery, right alongside other surgeons, residents, and researchers. The lab administrator put me through intensive training, teaching me the surgical ABC's—what the instruments were called, what they did, different types of sutures, how to make knots. In my life to that point, I'd cut open all of one frog, in biology class at Andover.

Three weeks after my training began, I was deemed ready to do transplants.

At first, I felt clumsy and pathetic. I put my thumb and index finger through the holes of the instruments so that I had a firm grasp of them, but it didn't feel natural. Gradually I got to see—got to *feel*—that if I covered the hole with my palm and exerted pressure with and through my palm, I could move faster and more dexterously. (This technique, called palming, I've employed in every surgery I have done since.) At first, I held the scalpel too far down the instrument and way too tightly—more rookie mistakes—but as I grew adept, I realized how lightly I could hold the scalpel, and how far up the shaft, and that doing so allowed for more sensitive touch.

Perhaps as important, the experience that summer gave me my first whiff—and I do mean *whiff*—of a rough-edge sensibility particular to many surgeons. One day, a pair of surgical residents operating on the beagles kindly offered to show me the intricate and fascinating anatomy of the aorta and vena cava.

"Hey, Cap, look at this," said one of them, leaning forward and urging me to join him for a closer look at the beagle's interior. He assured me it wouldn't hurt the dog because retractors were in place in the abdomen to keep the ribs spread apart.

I leaned forward for a look—at which point the other resident, who'd tiptoed behind me, shoved my face into the dog's abdomen.

I will never forget the stench of warm canine abdominal cavity.

I shot out of there, blood on my glasses and forehead and mask, and staggered back, head spinning.

"Welcome to the surgical corps," chided one of the residents, though I couldn't see which one.

I groaned weakly, teetering in the direction of a window, to replace the smell in my lungs with fresh Midwestern air.

Just then our supervisor walked in. He seemed to know right away what was going on—not that it took a genius. The scene—residents laughing; me, distressed, wiping blood off my glasses—was fairly self-explanatory.

"You boys are in big trouble," the supervisor warned the residents. Their laughter ceased immediately. Even in my fog I noted my surprise at how genuinely scared they looked.

My head had stopped spinning. I was no longer going to heave.

"We were just having some fun," I said, shrugging. The supervisor looked at me for a moment, expressionless, then walked out of the room. He never said a word about it.

When he'd gone, the residents smiled at me, grateful.

But I was the grateful one. I was just a kid, yet they'd initiated me into the medical fraternity, where both friendship and rivalry are unusually intense.

As to the kidney-transplant research: It was a spectacular triumph. We succeeded in showing that, at least in this breed of beagle, using cyclosporine as part of kidney transplants helped greatly in the acceptance of the new organs. A paper would be published about it, with Dr. Turcotte's name on top, and my name mixed in somewhere with the team's. Years later, the drug was approved for use in human kidney transplants, and a once risky procedure became fairly routine. Today, a kidney transplant involving a living donor has a *90+ percent* chance of success. Dr. Joseph E. Murray, the man from Massachusetts General Hospital and Brigham and Women's Hospital who had, a generation before, laid much of the foundation for all transplant surgery, would win the Nobel Prize for Medicine for his contribution—the only physician, amazingly, ever to win the prize.

The team's success was a perfect example of what I mean when I say scientific knowledge builds on previous knowledge to increase understanding and better people's lives.

Just as important to me back then, not one single beagle died during any of the surgeries that summer. Not one of those opened and closed by the surgeons or residents, or by me. My childhood dog, a blond Lab named Fresca, would have approved.

Thanks to Dr. Ransom, Dr. Turcotte, and the rest of the team, my decision to pursue medicine seemed vindicated. And I was grateful for the way they had included me, the youngest guy there. A kid never forgets who's been good to him.

For all my feeling for those men, though, I did not want to be a surgeon. I had decided on another branch of medicine, one that delighted my mother and thrilled my father.

I was going to be the world's greatest pediatrician.

I Don't Have
What It Takes

▼ ▼ ▼

*F*ocus and *drive*.

It's hard to find two words that describe better what it takes to become a successful surgeon.

Focus and *drive*.

It's what defined my last two years of college. I took all the premed courses I didn't take my first two years.

Senior year, I also managed to find the time, somehow, to fall in love for the first time. Victoria was a sophomore from New York City. Smart, intellectually curious, five feet eight, brunette, nicknamed Tory. We biked and played tennis. Our time together was always sweet. I knew that someday I wanted to be married, have kids, probably lots of them—not at all surprising for someone who came from a big family, and who has mostly happy childhood memories.

On graduation day, Tory was there. Life was perfect. But even greater joy lay just ahead.

The challenge of medical school.

It was at Duke Medical School that I learned how to be a doctor.

Sounds dumb, right? You go to medical school to learn how to be a doctor.

Except it doesn't always, or even often, work that way. Yes, of course medical school teaches you, in class and in clinical rotations, a basic fund of knowledge. Some concept of disease. Some concept of the treatment of disease. Medicines.

But to be a doctor, to really know how to care *for* patients rather than how to deal *with* them—that deep understanding may not happen at medical school. For me, I was fortunate already to have had a taste of it, by witnessing Dad's devotion and sense of rightness. The simple message of his coming home late so often—when I knew how much he loved his family—taught me that you can't ever turn off your responsibility to your patients. Ironically enough, his not being around—which had been the greatest deterrent when I was younger to my even considering a medical career—now revisited me as an important lesson to help prepare me for the difficulty, the *relentlessness,* of what I was about to embark on.

But as much as my father taught me, it was mostly secondhand observation: watching him through the car window as he made another house call; seeing him once every few months at the hospital; feeling his absence at home. (Later on, he became—and remains today, even in retirement—an even greater professional influence. Recently I phoned him with an immunology question that had stumped me. Dad knew the answer. It's pretty great having a man with a half century of medical experience always on call.)

My mentor at Duke, Dr. David Sabiston, taught me how to conduct myself, every day, as a healer of people. Like my father, he was devoted to his patients, worked hard, and stayed disciplined. But it was Dr. Sabiston's interaction with other doctors that was a revelation. I've never seen a superstar doctor—or any doctor, in fact—act so respectfully toward medical students, the indentured servants of our profession. If we med students did something wrong—and we were always doing something wrong—Dr. Sabiston would never admonish us publicly.

Yet he was stern. Each week during my rotation, one of us

had to review a case history of a patient and present it to the doctor, other med students, and some of the residents. The chief resident would prep us a bit, but mostly it was up to us to bone up on everything, to be armed to answer all questions about the history and management of the patient's disease. The presentations were made in one of the medical school libraries, a wood-paneled room decorated by photographs of previous chief residents, all of whom had obviously thrived at this kind of thing. The prize for a good presentation might be a phone call on your behalf, your final year of medical school—Dr. Sabiston calling the head of the medical residency program of your dreams and praising you to the stars. If you didn't do well? Let's not even consider that. *Maybe surgery is not right for you.* I was so nervous each time I presented to him, my knees actually knocked. I was grateful my lab coat covered the spectacle.

It was Dr. Sabiston who taught me probably the single most useful principle in my doctoring arsenal:

Do not treat without a diagnosis.

Again—sounds dumb, right? How *could* you treat without a diagnosis?

But the caution is more nuanced than that. It demands that, before you attempt to be a healer, you remember that first you're a *scientist.*

Sort out the problem. Think it through. Do not treat without a diagnosis.

You'd think every doctor would have learned this last tenet—or, if not, would have intuited it himself. But no. This fundamental notion (perhaps the doctor's equivalent to the lawyer's mantra to provide one's client with the best possible defense) is ignored and abused and forgotten by more doctors and hospitals than you want to know about. A few years ago, I got a call from a patient whose eyelids I'd lifted a year before. "This has nothing to do with plastic surgery, but I trust you," he said, his voice shaky. "I have prostate cancer." He then mentioned the name of a renowned New York–area hospital and said that they wanted to remove his prostate.

"How did they find the cancer?" I asked.

"Blood test," he said.

I hesitated a second. "Any tissue sample?"

"No, but a blood test."

"They're going to take out your prostate and possibly leave you incontinent without a tissue sample to verify that you have cancer?"

"See?" he said. "This is why I called."

He went back to the doctor and insisted a tissue sample be taken.

It was negative.

This happens all too frequently. A physician starts treating without having the proper diagnosis and ultimately injures, rather than helps, the patient. It's particularly infuriating because it's often so avoidable and delays real diagnosis.

Why does this happen? Are these doctors lazy? Intellectually undisciplined? I don't know. But every patient is entitled to a clear explanation of what is happening to him or her, why, how it's being treated, and why alternative treatments were rejected in favor of the one being followed. It's your body and your life, not to mention your peace of mind. Don't be afraid to ask for the explanation. If you still don't understand after it's been explained to you, then ask again, or ask more pointed questions. If your doctor can't explain clearly what's going on, then he or she doesn't understand the situation well enough. Get a new doctor.

In the end, Dr. Sabiston taught me only one thing, really. How to be a doctor.

I requested pediatrics as my first rotation.

Since Duke is a major cancer referral hospital—meaning it receives many of the most "complex" (read *terminal*) cases, largely from the southeastern United States—I saw dozens of children afflicted with cancer, some in infancy. Most of them suffered from leukemia or lymphoma. It's a sad euphemism but, in this role, Duke was termed a "tertiary medical center."

At the end of my first month in pediatrics, for whatever karmic reason, we received an unusually large influx of terminally ill children in a very short time—six in one week.

Of those, can you guess how many of them died by the following week?

Two?

One?

Four?

All of them. I saw every single one die.

When the sixth and last of those children died, I remember walking out of the hospital into the summer evening and taking a seat on the steps. I was more than just depressed. I was stunned, almost in shock, from what I'd just seen. I was literally dizzy with grief.

I couldn't see how I might spend the rest of my life witnessing the deaths of so many children; I simply couldn't. Of course, I could be a pediatrician and not work at a children's hospital that specialized in cancer. (It should be noted that, thanks to medical advances in the last generation, certain childhood cancers, particularly leukemia, have become far more treatable, at Duke and elsewhere. Duke was then and remains today one of the world's top pediatric cancer clinics.)

But it also seemed like running away. It seemed an acknowledgment that I could go only so far, no further. And that bothered me.

Bothered me? It destroyed me.

I was surrounded by Southern pine and dogwood, but the

trees that evening smelled like death. Everything did. Everything around me was dying. And everyone. I managed a bitter smile thinking that, from the moment I'd arrived on campus, death was lurking. On the first day of sign-up, I stepped up to the registrar and said brightly, "I'm here to enroll!"

The lady behind the desk looked up at me, quizzical and pained. "Have you heard? The King is dead."

"What?" I asked.

"Elvis died," said the registrar. "The King is dead."

What is wrong with me? I wondered now, sitting on the steps of Duke University Hospital.

I'm a doctor who can't handle death? Does this mean I'll make a rotten doctor, no matter which kind of medicine I go into?

What else is there for me to do?

Sadly, there was then, and remains now, a great need for young doctors to work in children's cancer hospitals. But there was just no way I would be one of the courageous men and women to do it.

My feeling of desolation, sitting alone on those steps, did not make me a rotten person, or even mean I would not succeed in medicine. I think I understood that. But it depressed me to think I didn't have it in me to be the doctor I'd hoped I could be.

Love Affair

▼ ▼ ▼

I never forget a face. Of all the faces I have laid eyes on in my life, hers may be the most unforgettable.

And when it was all over, I had fallen in love.

Use any of the clichés—struck by lightning, head over heels, shot through the heart—because they all apply. One day my life is heading in one direction. Sixteen hours later it's headed in a completely different, and absolutely unwavering, direction.

It happened at two in the morning, a sweltering July night in 1979, in Durham, North Carolina, in the trauma room of the ER, at Duke University Medical Center. Two surgeons and the ER staff were hunched and busy over a dying woman that night.

In saving one life, they also managed to transform a second one.

She was an all-American volleyball player. Earlier that night, the car that she and her boyfriend were driving had hit a tree. She flew through the windshield. She was spirited to the emergency room—and I do mean *spirited,* because not a person who saw her being rushed on a stretcher into the triage area in the ER expected her to survive the night. The ER team began to work on her, but the extent of the damage was historic. Her face, in particular, was crushed beyond recognition.

I knew nothing of all this. I was home, sleeping, dead tired from another night of medical school. I was three days into my newest rotation, surgery.

The phone rang. Bolting upright—a skill that after a while becomes reflex, once you give your life over to doctoring—I saw my alarm clock read just past 2:00 A.M.

"What?" I barked.

It was another intern, a friend on call that night at the hospital.

"Cap, man," he said with wonder in his voice. I was half-asleep, though, and couldn't detect anything besides an unwelcome wake-up call.

"I'm sleeping," I said.

"Get your ass over here," he said.

I threw on my pants and white coat and walked, bleary-eyed, the quarter mile to the hospital. In the all-American, five-foot-ten volleyball player, I witnessed the most devastated physical presence imaginable. Every major bone in her face was broken. Her eyes were dangling from their sockets, each one trying to peek into an ear. Every tooth was broken. Her nose was crushed in the middle. Her scalp was nearly torn off. She had multiple lacerations. Blood was everywhere. It was hard to determine what remained of her face, and if what was left could even be reconfigured as human anymore.

For the next sixteen hours—the first couple in the ER, the last dozen or so in the OR—I stood right beside a plastic surgeon and his resident and watched as they worked with a team of ophthalmologists and oral surgeons to reconstruct the woman's face. Calmly, and with ease, the surgeons used wire and high-speed drills to refit the bone back around her eyeballs. If the doctors were off by even one millimeter, they could blind her.

At one point during the surgery—we'd all lost track of time—the resident shook his head. "Hell of a way to make a living," he said gently.

The girl recovered.

I, however, would not. The next afternoon, when I finally walked out of the OR after a night of standing almost frozen, of no sleep, of staring intently for a dozen hours straight at this miracle of skill and medicine and care, I was not exhausted but exhilarated.

Plastic surgery!

A branch of medicine where you take a patient in some type of distress, and you make him or her significantly better . . . and you can actually see the immediate improvement? Just as powerful to me, though, was that it required such an impressive arsenal of abilities: concentration; physical dexterity and stamina; the intellectual alacrity to balance form and function; an awareness of aesthetics, structure, symmetry; a gift for understanding the human psyche and its frailties; compassion and candor and discretion.

(My initial love for the field, typical of most plastic surgeons, had nothing to do with cosmetic surgery. Our first exposure to the field is exclusively reconstructive surgery; observing and doing cosmetic surgery only comes later.)

After sixteen hours of watching a life and a face restored with the most amazing technical grace, I had found something that was miraculous for the individual patient, beneficial for society, and fulfilling for me. Plus, I felt—yes, deep in my bones—that I'd always had aptitudes that could now be exploited for just this pursuit: a love of aesthetics, a deeply visual memory. Even my ability to concentrate for hours at a time, honed while building models and sculpting clay as a kid because I was inept at sports, was now morphed into a virtue.

The day after watching the volleyball player return from the dead, I stood outside the medical school administrative office, waiting for the door to open so I could immediately change my course schedule for the coming year and focus on plastic surgery. Once I was done with that, I canceled all my vacation and holiday plans.

For the next two and a half years.

I finished the four-year program at Duke in three. I had high hopes. I was going to be a great plastic surgeon, like my mentors.

After what I had seen that summer night, a night that had unknowingly begun for me when a beautiful, athletic girl had hurtled through glass and struck a tree until she was shattered, only to be put back together again miraculously, there was no way in the world I could spend my life doing anything else.

My relationship with Tory consisted of our seeing each other every second or third weekend, alternating between Princeton and Duke. Among the med students, I was one of the few men in my class committed to a long-distance relationship. There was lots of romance between male and female doctors-to-be, and lots more young doctor and nurse couplings, too. Not that I needed to be spoken for to keep me from being distracted by the nurses and female residents. That it had become impossible for me to think of anything besides medicine should have been a tip-off to Tory, and to me, too, that making a relationship work would, now and for a long time to come, require me to be a very different person from the one I was becoming.

A few months into my surgical rotation I did my first appendectomy, as my professor stood across the table. It was the first time I'd made an incision into a living human being. This was not a sleeping dog or a cadaver. It was an out-of-body experience.

You pick up the scalpel, run it along the lower abdomen, and right away notice the particular pressure that must be exerted to open skin and expose the underlying tissue. Your fingers send messages to your brain, and vice versa, a feedback loop, so that you can adjust to this holy cow you have no clue what you're doing. No matter how much you have read or observed, nothing can compare to what you're going through now. There's nothing like the real thing.

Blood is coming out. I'm scared.

Do not look up at Dr. Young. He's right across the table watching you but you must focus on this, your fingers and brain working together, guiding you to go a little deeper.... Put your finger there,

Lesesne, that's it . . . any moment now you should be wetting your pants . . .

The more surgery I performed or assisted on, the more convinced I was that I wanted to be a plastic surgeon. Whereas my father got excited about the prospect of my being a doctor, and even more when I said I wanted to be a pediatrician, he was less thrilled about my decision to be a surgeon, and less so still about my being a plastic surgeon (though he would eventually come around). To me, plastic surgery offered an intellectual appeal that other types of surgery did not—the planning involved, the attention to detail, the fact that the entire body is the canvas, not just one organ. It's a younger surgical discipline, too, so a sense of discovery seemed more possible. Patients get well. They don't die. The aesthetic challenge appealed to me. I wanted to help people, to make their lives brighter. At this point I knew myself well enough to recognize that I did not have the emotional constitution to deal with what (for example) a cardiac surgeon must.

When my medical training at Duke ended, Dr. Sabiston—my mentor, the finest teacher I will ever know—offered me the chance to stay on as a resident. I'd learned so much at Duke, but I respectfully turned him down. I'd already been accepted as a surgical resident at Stanford, a top program. I treasured the doctor's offer as the penultimate compliment from him to me.

I say penultimate because he would pay me the *ultimate* compliment years later, when a woman showed up at my Park Avenue office to consult about a face-lift. When I asked how she'd heard of me, she said her longtime friend Dr. David Sabiston down in Durham had said I was the best.

As I left North Carolina, I hit the gas, breaking the speed limit in every state I crossed, so I could get to California as fast as I could and start being a surgeon.

Blood Everywhere

▼ ▼ ▼

June 20, 1980, I graduated from medical school. Two hours later I was speeding westward, all my belongings stuffed into my blue Datsun 310 hatchback. The trip took sixty hours. I slept in the car. As I crossed the middle of the country, rocketing toward my apprenticeship in one of the most prestigious surgical programs in the world, I thought:

I'm scared.

I don't know whether I'll make it through. Will I screw up? Will I kill somebody?

I rocketed past sights I'd never seen before, vistas that took my breath away—the Great Salt Lake, the Sierra Nevada—but as I neared California, I felt, mixed in with my excitement, a sense of solitude that bordered on loneliness. Out here under the big Western sky, I was far away from family and far from Tory, who had started law school in New York. Fair Acres Road and the leafy streets of Grosse Pointe were only a thousand miles behind me, but it might as well have been a thousand years.

I hinted to the surgery registrar—okay, more than hinted, *begged*—not to start me on the cardiac surgery unit. How about urology? No night call. An easy start. Just please don't make it cardiac, not to start with. I would have to cycle through cardiac at some point, I knew, just like every surgery resident, but it was legendarily awful—long hours, physically and psychologically demanding, the toughest rotation around. I was simply hoping for a little bit of time to adjust, maybe start with something a little less taxing. Even neurosurgery would have been a relief. I hadn't had a light week in three years.

They posted the schedule for all the first rotations.

LESESNE, CAP: CARDIAC.

One door closes. Another one opens.

So I wouldn't get a breather. But it was in the cardiac surgery rotation that I really learned to be a surgeon, and I suspect the same is true for most surgeons. That first month was the most intense, exhausting, frightening, chest-thumping of my life. I started out feeling stupid. Knowing nothing. Before getting too frustrated, though, I relied on all that solid Duke Medical School training to help me.

Sort out the problem. Think it through.

And then a funny thing happened: I *liked* cardiac. A lot. Having first dreaded it, I now found it so invigorating, and my surgeon mentors so likable and inspiring, that I thought I might become a cardiac surgeon. The team I worked under was first-rate: Several of them are chiefs of surgery at top hospitals across the country today. None was more encouraging to me, and on top of his game, than Norman Shumway. I worshiped him. My very first day on the job—June 28, a Saturday—I showed up for 6:30 A.M. orientation in my white coat. As I walked down the hall, Dr. Shumway approached and did something no one had ever done before.

He called me Dr. Lesesne.

At the orientation, we new guys were all told, repeatedly, that if we found ourselves in any kind of trouble or confusion, we were to call for help. That was the main lesson for the day. Otherwise, it was reasonable, even quiet. I left the hospital at 6:00 P.M.

Hey, this isn't too bad, I thought. Maybe cardiac wasn't always brutal.

The second day I was given something to do. A patient—a lawyer from Ogden, Utah, scheduled for a heart bypass the next day—had come in for his pre-op visit, and Dr. Shumway, busy with other patients, instructed me to "work up" Mr. Jensen—get his medical history and examine him (blood pressure, heart, lungs, etc.). But as soon as I walked into the examination room and explained to Mr. Jensen why I was there, he looked disgusted. Sensing how green I was, he insisted I fetch Shumway.

I obeyed, found the doctor, and brought him back to the exam room with me.

"Dr. Shumway," said Mr. Jensen, "I'm not letting some high school kid examine me."

I meekly opened the door and started to shuffle out, but Dr. Shumway put a firm hand on my shoulder. "Stay here, kid," he mumbled. I would learn that Dr. Shumway mumbled almost everything, in or out of the OR.

Dr. Shumway turned to the patient. "Mr. Jensen, Dr. Lesesne is my associate. If you don't let him examine you, I'm not operating on you. So if you're not up to being examined by him, you might as well get the hell out of my hospital, okay?"

"Okay," said Mr. Jensen.

"Good," mumbled Shumway, and gave me a pat. "So Dr. Lesesne will examine you, and I'll see you on the table tomorrow morning."

"Okay," said Mr. Jensen, nodding obediently.

In surgery, particularly cardiac surgery, there is no such concept as zero to sixty. You *start* at sixty, put the pedal to the floor, and leave it there. That's what happened during my very first operation at Stanford.

I was working under Dr. Shumway and Alex, his chief resident. A banker was getting a heart bypass. Such an operation is a big deal. Critical vessels to the heart are obstructed. People die.

The actual bypass—an unobstructed vein "harvested" from elsewhere on his body (in this case, his leg)—would be sutured on the outside of the heart, circumventing the obstruction.

In a few moments, we would be stopping the banker's heart and transferring pumping responsibility to a machine, while the doctors sutured vessels.

I was assigned to make an incision in the leg, starting at the inner groin and going down to the ankle. To free up the vein we wanted—the saphenous vein, which looks like a pipe with multiple branches—Alex cut all around it, then tied off the little branches leading out of it (called perforators). This stopped the bleeding. The saphenous is the perfect vein for a bypass: long, continuous, dispensable.

While Dr. Shumway placed tie-over sutures in the aorta to allow the bypass tube to be inserted, I began my lowly job of suturing up the skin on the leg. Alex occasionally glanced at me. In the last year of his residency, he was far more experienced than I.

"Dr. Shumway," the chief resident said casually, "he's screwing up the leg."

I'd left some gaps in the skin, which would require adding a few more sutures.

"We'll deal with it later," mumbled Shumway. "Duke guys are slow learners," he teased.

Surgical humor. Everything was going nicely.

Dr. Shumway lifted the patient's heart to get access to the left anterior descending artery. As I continued to sew, I heard Alex say, "Holy shit."

I looked up. Alex, whom I had always admired for his cool

demeanor, was frozen. His face was chalky, and his eyes, over his mask, had gone wide. I looked to see what he was staring at.

It must have been the blood pouring out of the patient's chest. A Vesuvius of blood.

There was a tear in the heart. The back wall of the heart had come apart when Dr. Shumway had gently lifted it to sew.

The patient was now bleeding and dying before everyone's eyes. I was frozen.

"What do we do now, chief?" Alex croaked.

"Alex," said Dr. Shumway, whose hands had not stopped moving, "this is what separates the men from the boys."

Blood was on the OR floor. Blood had soaked through the surgical towels surrounding the patient's chest. The patient had flatlined.

Dr. Shumway mumbled to switch the patient onto the bypass immediately, skipping normal preparatory steps such as checking the pump volume or asking about the readiness of the scrub tech—an OR assistant who had been with Shumway for years and probably knew the doctor's rhythms better than he did himself. Dr. Shumway had to assume that everything would work.

"Pump on," said Shumway.

The bypass pump whirred on. The bleeding stopped.

A machine was now pumping blood to the outer vessels of the patient's heart, although the amount needed to replace what had been lost was staggering.

Plus, the heart was still damaged. If it wasn't repaired soon, the patient would never leave the OR table alive.

Dr. Shumway called for a 4-0 prolene suture. The scrub tech had already slapped the right suture into the doctor's palm. Dr. Shumway, the smoothest surgeon I have ever seen, deftly began to repair the torn heart with the two prolene sutures. His fingers were moving fast, back and forth, back and forth, gently, sewing, tying off perforators. The concentration and skill were incredible. Alex and I stood motionless. Dr. Shumway's fingers kept moving.

Finally, they stopped. Shumway barked, "Vein."

Dr. Shumway took the vein he was handed, cut it for the right length, and performed a three-vessel bypass.

Once he completed this job, it was time to get the patient off the bypass machine and restart his heart. The doctor called for potassium and medication and now the paddles, and he was telling us all to stand clear so we didn't get electrocuted. He placed the paddles directly onto the patient's heart.

Boom!

Buh-bum. Buh-bum. Buh-bum.

The banker's heart was going again.

Dr. Shumway had no change in expression.

"Next case," he mumbled, and left the room.

Alex unfroze. He would go on to become one of the great heart surgeons in the Deep South.

One week later, the doors to Stanford University Hospital whooshed open and a banker—a leg vein now running from his proximal coronary artery to the base of his heart—walked out into the California sunshine.

My very first operation as a resident.

What's important in life?

To help people not die. That's one. But you see people die all the time. Old people, young people. Teenagers, pregnant women. There's no justice to it, no value system, no right, no wrong. They just die. Bad genes, bad luck. You don't know what to make of it. You've seen it happen like this before, in bulk, and then it involved children, lots of them. Do you get used to it? Does anyone? You were raised Anglican, went to Sunday school; throughout boarding school and college you attended church. You're not sure what you believe. You've read the Bible, the Torah, the Koran, the Bhagavad Gita.

People keep dying.

When you see death day after day, you have to do something positive with it. You help people, yes. Well, that's good. Keep them from dying too soon. Keep them from living with sickness, from living too unhappily. Good.

But what about for yourself? How do you keep from losing it? How do you keep despondency at bay?

You cultivate a healthy appreciation that every day is special. You appreciate that every day may also be your last.

Welcome to the life of a medical resident, cardiac rotation.

Tory, my girlfriend of five years and in her first year of law school at New York University, said she wanted to get married.

I told her I wasn't ready.

We broke up.

A year later, she would marry someone else.

Nasty Surgeons, Not Enough Sleep, and Other Myths

▼ ▼ ▼

A t Stanford, as at all surgical residency programs, my plastic surgery rotation consisted almost entirely of work and training in reconstructive, not cosmetic, surgery—hand surgery, head and neck reconstruction, postorthopedic-surgery reconstruction to cover exposed implants. Later, I would need to learn the nuances of cosmetic surgery, of course; I couldn't expect to really understand spatial dimensions, 3-D relationships, skin thicknesses, and anatomical planes until I'd done more face-lifts than I could count.

But I was in my surgical residency, first and last, to learn what it takes simply to be a good surgeon.

Watching and working with great surgeons, I was learning what their common traits were. They were decisive. (Outside the OR, surgeons are often reflective and even filled with self-doubt; in the OR, they're decisive.) When a problem arose, there was no dithering. Before you blinked, they were already working toward a solution, or taking a different approach. Their hands were always moving. They knew the ins and outs of the procedures and they were technically skilled, of course, but, of equal importance, they had a suppleness and resourcefulness of mind to take a different course. Like great chess players, the most skilled ones had plotted their actions several moves in advance. Over the years, watching them at Michigan, Duke, Stanford, and several New York hospitals (among others), I have always marveled at and appreciated the great ones.

You could say they're hyperconfident and sure of themselves. Cocky and arrogant, even. You almost can't help being that way. First, surgery tends to attract the most alpha, testosterone-fueled of an already alpha group, doctors. (Of the twenty-four plastic surgical residents in my six-year program at Stanford, three were women. I don't know how much of the scarcity of female surgeons is systemic bias, how much is self-selection, how much is other factors.) Second, what we do is pretty mind-blowing, if you think about it. Every once in a while, while operating, I'll catch myself thinking about how odd, how unnatural, it is to do what I do: *I'm taking a knife to someone, she's bleeding, there's her fat, there's her muscle* . . . In my first weeks during my plastic or otolaryngology surgery rotations at Stanford, when I might be operating on patients with cancers, my momentary, out-of-body ruminations were even more sobering: *His life is in my hands. . . . If I screw up, he could be seriously injured . . . or I could kill him. . . .* It's a weird, unique, complicated, *ultimate* thing we surgeons do.

Confidence entered me sometime after I'd done a thousand of a given procedure. To me, confidence simply means an awareness that I've put in the work, that I know my abilities and limitations, that I appreciate medicine is both a science and an art, that I've done all I reasonably can to protect the patient and myself against the unpredictable.

I have also watched surgeons who shouldn't be surgeons. They delay. They are unprepared. Often, they're the cockiest of all. (Unlike the rest of us, they're not constantly terrified that something might go wrong.) When you think you know everything, you don't train as hard. Or you get sloppy. I know of a self-righteous, quick-to-pontificate chief of surgery who felt he didn't need to be in the OR in the moments before performing a hernia repair—a common, generally uncomplicated operation. Instead he was drinking coffee in his office while his thirteen-year-old patient was being anesthetized. The anesthesiologist, alone in the OR, lost control of the patient's airway. While inserting the endotracheal tube (for breathing), the anesthesiologist couldn't quite see where it was going. A laryngeal spasm ensued and the patient's oxygen level dropped, initiating a disastrous sequence that culminated in the boy's cardiac arrest and death. Had the surgeon been in the OR, he could have performed an emergency tracheotomy, something all licensed surgeons learn our first year as interns.

The thoughtful doctor, on the other hand, the one who knows the stuff cold but also realizes his or her limitations, tends to train harder, tries continually to learn, and is willing to entertain a wider range of treatment possibilities (and is more likely to treat *you,* not the symptoms). Because the thoughtful doctor prepares better, he's more likely to pick up mistakes *before* they manifest themselves, thus avoiding them. In what amounts to an irony, then, the more modest doctor, the one who can imagine his own fallibility, will probably end up being regarded as *more* infalliable by grateful patients and staff than are doctors who ooze self-assurance.

There were several surgical and medical myths whose truth (or not) I was beginning to sift through. For example:

Surgeons are emotionally detached, even nasty.

Largely false—except for surgeons who specialize in cancers and *are* notoriously cold, not because they're innately misanthropic but because they see so many people die. It's a well-circulated opinion among surgeons that urological surgeons are easily the nicest among surgeons, and cardiac the most intense. Plastic surgeons are often called the "fairy surgeons"—mostly because our surgery is more aesthetic and largely elective, and non-life-threatening. We're more artistic. And there tend to be, by my observation, more gay surgeons in plastic surgery than in other surgical disciplines.

Surgeons, particularly plastic surgeons, are in it for the money.

Some are, of course; most are not. It's simply too brutal a life to do it primarily for the money. Dan Baker, a well-known New York plastic surgeon, told me he works harder now, in his mid-sixties, than he's ever had to work before. We see each other walking to the local Starbucks at 6:30 A.M. on a Sunday—and that's *after* we've seen our patients.

A nice office suggests a successful practice and a good doctor.

Plastic surgeons in particular are guilty of turning their offices and waiting rooms into palaces (gorgeous fish tanks, flower collections), often because they feel that their wealthy clientele expect it. Dr. Joseph Murray, a brilliant surgeon and the only physician ever to win the Nobel Prize for Medicine, had benches in a hall outside his modest office.

If a surgeon does lots of operations a day, he must be good.

Volume is not indicative of quality. There's a balance between being quick and facile, on one hand, and really understanding the operation, on the other. When surgeons routinely take longer than usual to complete standard operations, it probably means they're not as sure and prepared as they should be. I've heard women boast about how their plastic surgeon took seven and a half painstaking hours to do a face-lift, suggesting that he was especially careful. To me it suggests he's probably not very good. The best plastic surgeons are neither too fast nor too slow.

*The number of papers published or prestigious titles
(e.g., department chair, medical society president) suggests
a good doctor.*

Not necessarily. In fact, there may be an inverse relationship. I have
met several surgeons who published papers so often, they scarcely
performed surgery anymore. That might not be a doctor you should
go to.

Good doctors know a lot.

No—and yes. That is, we *do* know a lot—but about very, very little,
and that area of expertise narrows over time, for two reasons: One,
doctors get older and more experienced; two, the field of medicine
becomes ever more specialized. I have come to know a great deal
about the face, millimeter by millimeter, but less and less about hand
surgery, a specialty that I, as all plastic surgeons, was trained in.

*Residents (and interns and medical students) are so sleep-
deprived it compromises their ability and particularly their
judgment.*

Myth—not that they're sleep-deprived, but that they can't function
on little sleep. People make too much of this one. Yes, you can be exhausted and your thought processes change, but you compensate.
When you work in a hospital, you cope. I've never failed in a case
because I was tired, and God knows, as a resident I operated tired.
You teach yourself to recognize when you're too depleted. Hospital
training is excellent for teaching residents that at the slightest sign
of uncertainty, they should *always seek backup*. Or delay the procedure. Because this idea was beaten into my brain for years, now, in
private practice, if I've been operating all day, and I don't feel well

or alert, and another operation awaits, I know to reschedule. Patients understand. As for being on your feet operating and concentrating sometimes for five, seven, ten, even sixteen hours at a time: It's not a problem. You're so focused on the patient and what you need to do, the body and mind transcend fatigue.

These are just a few lessons I've learned in medicine.

The invasive cancer had wrapped around the patient's left carotid artery, threatening to slowly reduce the blood flow to the brain—in essence, to strangle it. (The left and right carotids are the two main arteries to the brain.) If I was one millimeter off, I would puncture the carotid, which would cause massive, rapid, gushing bleeding, and I would wipe out half his brain, paralyzing or killing him.

To get control of the cancer, I worked around the normal tissue to get at the abnormal tissue. I removed the left maxilla—the cheekbone—only to find that the tumor had invaded the back of *that*. I kept dissecting tissue, sending it to the pathology lab, and results kept returning with the phrase *positive margins*—that is, the cancer was continuing to show up. Without getting a result of *clear margins,* the patient would die.

I had yet to find the end of the cancer's incursion. I removed the patient's whole left face (essentially) to see that the tumor had infiltrated all the way to the base of his brain. I started going deeper, millimeter by millimeter, using scissors to cut away soft tissue, a drill with a bur when I needed to shave bone.

You know, if I screw up at all, I thought, *this will be very, very bad. I will kill him.*

Finally, I got a pathology result of clear margins.

I leaned back. This was much bigger than I had anticipated. Now I had to close the hole in his face.

How the hell was I going to do that?

My thoughts raced through what plastic surgeons call "the reconstructive ladder." The first option is simply to close the skin. I couldn't do that here because too much was missing.

The second option is to apply a skin graft, usually taken from the leg. I couldn't do that either, because the skin graft wouldn't take to bare bone, and he was missing too much tissue.

The third option is a flap—which means to rotate skin, fat, and usually muscle from somewhere else on the body. In his case, I decided on a delto-pectoral flap from the chest.

Eventually, a couple short years after feeling inept, after having no confidence as a surgeon, I'd found it. Over time and numerous procedures, especially more complicated surgeries, I'd found it. Mentors covered me less and less. The responsibility and complexity of what I was given to do kept growing. No longer was I doing an appendectomy or taking out a superficial lipoma. One day I realized simply that *I* was now the one with the high-speed drill in my hands, *I* was the one screwing plates on to close a fractured cheekbone, millimeters from the eye. One slip and *I* was the one who would puncture the eye and blind him.

With each pass of the drill, I moved faster, smoother, totally in control. I was no longer scared.

In the 1980s, the Bay Area was a hotbed for sex-change surgery, and I operated on transsexuals at Stanford. Only I didn't know it. At least not the first time she—he—was under my care.

Mary Lou came to the Stanford Clinic with an infected breast implant. She was the first breast implant patient I'd ever seen. I looked at her in the examination room, with an attending resident present. Mary Lou described her problem. I prescribed antibiotics and told her we'd probably need to replace the implant.

As I walked down the hall afterward, a group of senior residents surrounded me, laughing.

"Clueless," said one.

"What?" I said.

"What'd you think of Mary Lou?" one of them asked me.

"What do you mean?"

"Well," said one of them, "would you ever date her?"

"Huh?"

"Would you date him?" said another.

"What are you talking about?" I asked.

"Cap," said the first, "exactly how clueless are you?"

Very. Had they not chided me, I would never have known that she was in fact a he, probably in the final stages of sexual reassignment, prepenectomy.

The more senior residents would play a joke on interns. We'd all go to a Palo Alto bar popular among many groups, including postoperative transsexuals. The residents would buy a few beers for the intern, then elbow him to hit on one of these great-looking women—and some of them were truly great-looking. The poor intern was as clueless in that trannie bar as he was his first time in an OR.

In fairness to the residents, they always yanked the intern away before things went too far.

At least, that's what I was told.

Our parotid glands are just in front of and below our earlobes. They secrete saliva into our mouth. For the plastic surgeon, they are particularly important because they wrap around the nerves that move the muscles of the face.

The attending surgeon, nurse, patient, and I were in the Veterans Hospital in Palo Alto. Millimeter by millimeter, I was removing a superficial (closest to the skin surface) lobe of the parotid, a gland full of invasive cancer. All surgery requires concentration, of course, and can turn disastrous if one misses by the slightest amount—too deep, too far right, too far left. But this operation was more than usually treacherous. Total and permanent facial paralysis awaited just this side of a mistake.

The attending surgeon walked out for a moment, and it was left to me to dissect out the nerve away from the tumor. I was focusing as hard as I possibly could; still, I sensed something weird going on, though I hardly registered what. . . . Had the table just hopped? Was I trembling? Was I more exhausted than I thought? Physically, emotionally? No, I felt fine, or thought I did. Sure, I was tired, if I stopped to think about it, but fine. I was a twenty-six-year-old surgical resident, more adroit and getting smoother, at Stanford University Medical Center. I just needed the OR nurse to hand me the iris scissors for delicate dissection.

I continued to cut, concentrating on the nerves and the gland immediately before me. Things proceeded smoothly. I dissected the nerve free from the gland.

I took a breath and stepped back, rewarding myself a moment to recalibrate.

The table was not moving. Perhaps I'd hallucinated the whole thing.

"That was very odd," I said, and looked up at my nurse.

Behind her, a giant crack ran down the wall.

According to the nurse, the earthquake had lasted close to two minutes.

Neither romance nor a social life were even options at this point. I was too locked into my training. I was soaking in everything I could from the great surgeons around me.

After assisting one of my plastic surgery mentors on a face-lift, he pulled off his gloves and shared with me one of the amusing little secrets of a cosmetic procedure that succeeds *too* well.

"The big joke, Cap," he said, "is that when you do enough of these and you get really good, you start thinking of what we do as 'anti-Darwinian.' We're changing physical appearance, the natural expression of the genes. Make someone look *too* good, and they start to forget that that's not what they really look like. Then she marries, has a child—and suddenly the baby emerges and he's ugly. Big eyes, funny nose, giant ears."

He looked almost satisfied to visualize the moment of realization for the new mother.

"We're not changing the insides, Cap," he said.

I was doing cardiac surgery at the VA Hospital. I'd been up since six that morning, on rounds by seven, had completed three open-heart procedures that day. Now it was six thirty at night and I was walking down the center aisle of the CCU, my white coat covering my blood-spattered scrubs, my stethoscope banging at my side. I was adjusting lines, IVs, and meds for my patients. Five beds down each side, ten direly sick patients total, all hoping (if they were conscious) to get out of that big green room alive; their families in the waiting room or scattered about the city or country praying that their loved ones would get well.

As in most any cardiac care unit, there was the relentless beep-beep of ventilator bags, the drips going, the IVAX machines, the EKGs measuring everyone's extremely precarious heart activity. Whenever you're in a place like that, even if you've been around it for a while, there's always a seed in your brain—sometimes big, sometimes small—but always there:

Thank God I'm okay. At least that's not me.

I moved to check on my next patient, a post-bypass being tended to by a nurse. She had adjusted his IV line. I told her I wanted to put in an A-line (an arterial line, to measure the blood's oxygen) and she nodded. Then she looked past me, as something over my shoulder caught her attention.

I turned to see what she was staring at. The TV over the bed of the patient behind me.

On the TV screen, amid all the steady drip-drip of the IVs, an incredibly dreamy scene played out. At least one patient's TV was always on in the ward, and it was usually just white noise to me. But now the TV was delivering something miraculous, and what it was showing seemed to be moving almost in slow motion. On-screen, two people walked gracefully down an aisle, he in a long morning coat, she in the most spectacular wedding dress, a train that must have been ten yards long, all silk and shimmering jewels. They stepped into a carriage. It was right out of a fairy tale.

Actually, it *was* a fairy tale.

The nurse moved to turn up the volume.

"And here is the new Princess of Wales meeting her subjects for the first time," the announcer purred in an erudite British accent, as Prince Charles, future king of England, and his new bride, Princess Diana, began to wave at the adoring crowd from their carriage. She radiated beauty.

Youth, love, future. Here I was, among men and women who would be grateful for a brief, highly medicated, not too painful future.

I wiped my brow with a sleeve of my blood-covered scrubs, then began to insert an A-line into the radial artery of the sickly man's hand, to keep tabs on his blood gases.

New York Practice

▼ ▼ ▼

After three thrilling, exhausting, mind-bending years at Stanford, I came East for another residency, this one specializing in plastic surgery, at Cornell and New York Hospital, another world-renowned institution. In North Carolina I'd learned to be a doctor, in California a surgeon. In New York, I would learn to be a plastic surgeon.

At New York Hospital, I learned an enormous amount—about different types of face-lifts, about rhinoplasties, about dealing with burns. At Sloan-Kettering Cancer Center, one of my last rotations, I did reconstructive surgery on cancer patients. As a surgeon doing that kind of work your mind-set is very different from what it is when you do cosmetic work. You're not worried at all about scars. Instead, you're doing things like repairing large defects and covering chest holes. You're happy if the patient is just able to leave the hospital alive.

I also learned who some of the good guys in New York medicine were, and who were the bad guys.

When that two-year plastic surgery residency at Cornell came to a close, I had two professional options: to apprentice with an older plastic surgeon (if I could land such a job), or go out on my own. I decided on the latter.

I thought I was ready to take on the world, nervy as that was. I was young, unknown, knew almost nothing about how the business worked, had no patients, and was unfamiliar with the rank and file of the Manhattan upper crust, where so many patients would eventually come from.

Other than that, I was set to go.

My last day as a resident at New York Hospital, I was nervous but excited about my future. I felt like a runner in the starting blocks. It was a gorgeous, late-spring day in Manhattan. A tall woman in a black Danskin top, red leather skirt, and tights passed me and entered the exam room. My last patient as a resident! Because I knew I would not be operating on her, I told the brand-new resident to "work her up"—take her basic info and do a standard physical exam—after which I would come in and sign off on the proposed surgery.

Two minutes later, the resident came to fetch me.

"She wants to see you," she said.

I recalled my own virgin exam-room debacle, at Stanford years earlier, when, as the new resident there, the patient had sneered at having "some high school kid" examine him.

I was all set to make my own protect-the-dignity-of-the-new-resident speech to the tall lady in the leather skirt and the Danskin top. But when I walked into the exam room and smiled at her, something clicked immediately.

To start, she had awfully large ankles.

I whispered to the young resident that I would take this one, not to worry, and closed the door, leaving me alone in the room with the patient. I smiled and introduced myself.

"Dr. Lesesne," she said in a deep voice, "I wanted to speak to a man."

I nodded.

"I'd like to have breast implants," she said, then paused.

I waited a moment to see if more was coming.

"I want them put on my back," she said.

Because I'm Midwestern-slow, it was only now that I was getting that she was a he.

You'd think all that time I'd put in on transsexual cases at Stanford would have sharpened my eye, and I would have picked up on it when she—he—first passed me on her way to the exam room. Especially with those large ankles.

"Breast implants on your back," I repeated.

"Yes," he boomed. "So my lover can have something to hold on to when he and I have sex."

It took a moment to get the visual, and it might take you a moment, too, so here:

Man dresses like a woman. His lover is a man. But the lover—a gay man—wants breasts to hold on to while he's having sex with our man, so he can imagine he's having sex with a woman.

Ergo, this patient's breast implants need to be on his back.

Check.

"Got it," I said.

Because it was my last day, and he was my last-ever patient as resident, I felt in a puckish mood. I decided to refer him to an attending doctor who had always been a jerk to all of us residents.

"I don't do that particular operation," I told the gay transvestite, "but if you'll go right now to this doctor"—I scribbled down the irritating surgeon's name and Fifth Avenue office address, knowing who would be in his waiting room—"he may be able to help."

It was mean, I confess. The darker side of medical humor.

An hour later, the nurse told me that the doctor to whom I'd sent the transvestite was on the phone. As soon as I put my ear to the receiver, he was spewing.

"*Whichoneofyougoddamngeniusessentthisqueentodisruptmy office?!*"

As much as I loved the teamwork and camaraderie of working with other doctors, it was time for me to go solo.

At least until I had business cards made up.

▼

It was a bold move, and not the best one. I could have—should have—stayed on a few more years at New York Hospital, getting more experience, handling a variety of cases, establishing my name as a plastic surgeon, and not worrying about paying my bills. Even better, I should have apprenticed with an established surgeon and learned the business from him. I could have met his patients, observed how he interacted with them, and learned medical and practical aspects of running an office.

I didn't have patients or patience.

I was so anxious about succeeding in New York on my own, for weeks I went nearly sleepless. *How am I going to make it here?* I wondered. I found a Park Avenue office I could share with a group of older doctors, but they were constantly screwing me: They'd tell me I could have the OR for this time slot or that one—then, at the last minute, they'd inform me there'd been a change and that *they* needed the OR then. It made me look unprofessional to the few patients I did have.

One Saturday morning at six thirty, the phone rang. (I knew, by the hour, that it had to be another surgeon calling.) It was Dr. Sherrell Aston, one of New York's most well-respected plastic surgeons, calling to say that Manhattan Eye, Ear & Throat Hospital, where he was an attending surgeon, had an opening for a fellow and would I be interested in joining them?

A pretty great bolt from the blue. Just the phone call I was looking for. It seemed the proverbial answer to a prayer.

But independence pulled at me. Before I could say yes to him, I had to think about it. I thanked Dr. Aston for his generous offer and told him I'd call him after the weekend.

Monday I called to thank him again. And to turn it down.

Who says you learn from your mistakes?

Only later did I find out that Dr. Aston was possibly interested in taking me on as a partner, after a few years. He was thirteen years my senior and highly regarded by doctors and patients all over the city. We would have gotten along, I was sure. I knew how to be a team player.

If I had said yes to him, or joined another plastic surgeon, it might have shaved years off my time line for making it in New York. On the other hand, I wasn't going to waste time second-guessing my decision. If my persistence and impatience had driven me to this point, at age thirty, then it was inevitable that those traits would cause me to take some wrong turns, too. I'd been trying for so long to get into the wider world, from the moment I'd left my small, leafy Michigan suburb to find excitement in the East, in a different and, to me, more intriguing world.

Still, the go-it-alone route I was now taking would be the tougher one by far.

The first step was getting hospital privileges. I got them at two places—Manhattan Eye, Ear & Throat Hospital and Beekman Downtown. I now had ORs to use for my own patients, especially useful if my office partners continued to pull the rug out from under my OR time. My hospital affiliations also meant I would get work by being on their ER call list. If someone came into the ER requiring plastic surgery, I'd be one of the surgeons to get the call. I'd get paid if the patient had insurance; if he or she didn't, which was half the time, well, then I'd just done surgical pro bono work.

One of my big problems was that I wasn't a self-promoter. I didn't know a good way to announce that I was officially open for business. (Today, lots of plastic surgeons advertise everywhere— *New York* magazine, *Texas Monthly, L.A. Confidential,* infomercials, radio.) I was confident I could do good surgery. But how would I find enough patients to operate on? So that I would eventually have enough business to run my own Park Avenue practice?

I was broke and unknown in New York, a plastic surgeon with barely a practice. I had no clients. I was invisible to everyone.

I knew that if I worked constantly and stayed the course, it would work out, but this time, seriously, I had bitten off more than I could chew.

Years later, after I had established myself with many friends and patients, I started to take the occasional three-day weekend. Once every two or three months, I would fly out on Delta Airlines on a Friday evening from JFK to Atatürk Airport, in Istanbul, Turkey, hail a cab to the downtown Swiss Hotel, shower, eat breakfast, and then see consults until eight that evening, go out with friends for dinner overlooking the Bosphorus—the magical strait that cuts through the city, dividing Europe from Asia—maybe go to a coffee club until midnight, get a good night's sleep, see more patients the next day, then fly back to New York Sunday night.

On one trip, I decided to throw a cocktail party for my many close Turkish friends. But I had to be careful about whom I invited: I couldn't include everyone I wanted to because I'd operated on quite a few of them, and they might feel as if to attend the party would be to "out" themselves. But there were enough close friends to choose from, and in many cases I'd gotten to know several generations of families—parents, grandchildren, etc. I hosted it at the Cirgon Palace, by their gorgeous reflecting pool, overlooking the Bosphorus.

My strong connection to this beautiful and fascinating country had been sparked years before, when two well-to-do, already stunning Turkish women came to me for eyelid lifts. Happy with their results, they recommended me to their friends. The parade of attractive Turkish women through my office was almost laughable: They were routinely dark-haired, green-eyed beauties, gracious, well-mannered, and intelligent. Some could have drowned in the amount of jewels and Chanel they owned. Soon I had a flourishing minipractice just among Turks, women and men both. In the beginning, they came to my Park Avenue office (world travelers and international businesspeople, they frequently passed through New York or even maintained homes here), but I would often go to Turkey for consults. I'd been to Istanbul roughly thirty times and had gotten to know the city quite well. I especially loved the art and architecture. Because of the numerous friendships I'd developed there, I had even read the Koran, so I could understand their nuances. Turkish women, in particular, tend to communicate elliptically. "Oh, Cap," they would often say to me, "you know what I mean." It was imperative that I understood what, in fact, they meant.

The party I threw was about friendship, not plastic surgery, especially considering the covert nature of my business; many of the people there didn't even know I was a surgeon, much less a plastic surgeon. They knew I was American, a New Yorker, a doctor. A beautiful crowd came. Their money had come from concrete, banking, cars, real estate, steel, textiles, and telecom. There were multimillionaires and high-ranking government officials. I think everyone had a grand time.

Kemal—the brother of a friend of mine—came over and toasted me on this festive night.

"A very special evening, my good friend," he said, and took a sip of champagne. Then his look turned curious. "Every time my wife comes back from New York, she looks better. What do you do again?"

"I'm a doctor," I said.

"What kind of doctor?"

"A surgeon."

"What kind of surgeon?"

"Plastic surgeon."

He nodded, sipped his champagne, then raised his glass in

toast once more. "Now you really are my good friend," he said, smiling underneath his mustache. *"Inshallah."*

"Inshallah," I said. *If God wills it.*

One of my friends, an heiress named Melek, said that the next evening she was going to a party in Gstaad and asked me to join her. After a morning of consults, I drove to the airport for a Turkish Airlines flight to Geneva, where a limo met us. We wound our way to a castle in the Swiss Alps, where a party was being hosted by Umberto II, heir to the throne of Italy. Surrounding me were displaced European royalty. Also present was the legendary Brazilian plastic surgeon, Ivo Pitanguy, who was flirting with all the women. Afterward, Melek and I walked the streets of Gstaad. I paused to look at a surprisingly inexpensive watch in the window of a jewelry store. Melek, who had been looking elsewhere and had kept walking, turned to see where I was. She doubled back, and now she herself was taken by something in the jewelry store window—a huge diamond necklace, with emeralds in the center, and matching emerald earrings. She entered the store.

Fifteen minutes later, she exited, with the necklace, the earrings, and most of the remainder of the window display (though not the cheap watch I'd been eyeing and had decided not to buy).

Two and a half million dollars in jewels. In nine hundred seconds.

But that sort of episode would happen much later.

For now, I was still getting stiffed half the time after I performed surgery in the ER. My notion of a glamorous evening was dining alone at the local French restaurant. And the only journey I cared about was the one that led to my becoming a surgeon, a good one, in New York.

You Can't Go Home Again

▼ ▼ ▼

What bothered me most the summer of 1986 is that the goal I was shooting for—a private plastic surgery practice in New York City—was not happening. Too expensive. Not enough contacts. Not enough contacts in the right world.

Fortunately, there was a place I could go that was *not* too expensive, where I had lots of contacts, and where I had lots of contacts in the right world—in short, I could make my dream of a private practice come true immediately.

Grosse Pointe, Michigan.

The fear of practicing in New York had sent me home. But when I left the city, I didn't look at it as a surrender. I knew I would return.

My parents were thrilled to have me back: I'd been gone, basically, for seventeen years, since I was fourteen. And I didn't have to look hard to find my medical digs: I would share my father's office on Mack Avenue, in Grosse Pointe. Within ten days, I was booked up, largely because my father's name carried such respect in town. I had invaded the turf of the handful of plastic surgeons in the area, and they were not happy about the development. But that was too bad: Wherever you practice, it's going to be competitive—maybe even more so with elective surgery, where people can take their time choosing whom they want. I would be grabbing lots of my new patients from the upper middle class and working class of Detroit. It would be a broad-based practice. Getting hospital privileges wouldn't be a problem. And it didn't hurt that my educational background was first-rate. (I may not have been a natural self-promoter but I knew enough that Duke Medical School, Stanford surgical residency, and Cornell and New York Hospital plastic surgery residency were big pluses.)

This was going to work, I thought.

Even better, a woman that all of us boys had noticed as teens (she was twenty when I'd left for Andover) was still in Grosse Pointe, and just as attractive as ever. Chris had been an all-state swimmer all those years ago, and she was still athletic—five feet ten, swimmer's build, a blue-eyed brunette.

We met at a country club party, and suddenly she noticed me; I was no longer a fourteen-year-old Poindexter to her twenty-year-old vision of loveliness. Older and wiser and more confident now—and reasonably within age range, thirty-two to her thirty-eight—I asked her out to dinner, and she agreed. Later, we went sailing and biking together. She worked for the local newspaper, the publishing side. For two months during that summer, while I was finding the rhythm of being a plastic surgeon on my own, Chris and I enjoyed a lovely romance. In a way, it was like *Summer of '42,* only better. I was not the teenage boy who gets one night with Jennifer O'Neill; I was the teenage boy a decade and a half later who gets Jennifer O'Neill to take him seriously.

I was doing surgery, which I loved. I was learning how to run a business, which I needed. And I was enjoying my evenings with a swell, pretty girl.

Maybe perfection *was* attainable.

It lasted for only a moment.

Returning to Michigan was a failure. Within weeks of being back, I realized that Thomas Wolfe was right: You can't go home again. I loved being close to my parents, but I'd been gone too long. I had changed. I'd seen the world. Instead of being comfortable at home, I was nervous. Every day there, I missed being in the thick of New York activity.

Even Chris would not be enough to keep me in Grosse Pointe.

I had put in too many years of medical training, and I knew I had to give everything to that, wherever it needed to take me, before I could concern myself with other parts of my life.

Chris understood. We promised to stay in touch, no strings attached.

At the end of August, two months into my Michigan practice, I left my dad's office on Mack Avenue. The other plastic surgeons in the area, I'd like to think, were glad to see me go. Years later, one of them came up to me at a party. "I'd have paid your ticket," he said. I flew back East. I was going to try it there if it killed me.

Back in New York, I was driven. I was not going to fail. I still had to rent office space; I was as broke as I'd been at the beginning of the summer. I didn't hear from Chris for months and assumed she'd moved on; I admit I didn't take time to call her either. I figured we would see each other the next time I was home.

I continued to cover work in the ERs, looking for referrals. I rented office space in Westchester County, too, north of the city, and became affiliated with the hospital nearby, so that I could expand my base; it was dumb to rely for my livelihood exclusively on Manhattanites, millionaires or otherwise. There was no time to go home for Christmas. I called Chris.

Her line had been disconnected.

I continued to drive forward. Almost all my work was reconstructive, typical for a plastic surgeon starting out. Occasionally I removed small skin cancers.

Finally, I got my first-ever cosmetic surgery patient of my own.

Clara Lee, a meek lady in her midfifties, came to my office. She said that I had done some reconstructive work on a friend of her daughter's and did I do face-lifts?

Yes, I told her eagerly.

When it was time to pay me, she took out a brown paper bag

and removed a fat bunch of $20 bills and gave me the proper amount.

Two years later, two FBI agents showed up at my office, a man and a woman. They asked me questions about a Clara Lee—did I know her?

"Yes," I said.

"What do you know?" the male agent asked while the female agent snooped around the room.

"I did a procedure on her," I said.

"A face-lift?" he asked.

"Yes."

"Do you have any before and after photos of her?"

"Actually, I don't. She didn't want me to take any pictures of her afterward."

The male agent nodded. The female agent was now studying my diplomas hanging on the wall.

"Why all these questions?" I wanted to know.

"Clara Lee was a branch manager of Citibank who embezzled two million dollars and then fled to South America. We've been trying to track down leads of her whereabouts."

I nodded, stunned, and the agents soon left.

Maybe one minute later, there was a knock on the door and the female agent entered. She closed the door behind her. She was maybe thirty-five.

"Do you do breast implants?" she whispered.

Things slowly but steadily began to pick up. I did an arm liposuction for an outgoing forty-six-year-old woman who was happy enough to come back for liposuctions of her saddlebags (outer legs) and abdomen. She told me she loved going out to bars and she loved men, but she felt uncomfortable sleeping with them because of her stomach. Months later, she returned and pointed to her thighs and stomach. "Can you believe how lean I am?" She told me her sex life had improved. "Men look at me differently."

I did a face-lift on a patient without using sedation, a pretty rare occurrence. (I used only local.) But he wanted it that way: He was an actor in Alcoholics Anonymous, and he felt that being sedated was breaking his vow. It was strange having him look up at me while I was doing surgery, and far stranger still for me to be conversing with the patient during the operation.

The OR was my (and any surgeon's) favorite place in the world. It's where I was in total control. As someone at Stanford had said, a surgeon's first love is the OR, his second is his patients, his third is sex.

Consumed by work, when I looked up, it was springtime in New York, the trees blooming. I was finally getting more referrals. It was no longer so far-fetched to think I might truly realize my dream of being a surgeon. I was thirty-three.

I finally had a chance to call a friend from home. I asked if he knew where Chris had moved to.

"Moved?" he asked. "She died."

Two months after I had left Grosse Pointe, the friend told me, Chris was diagnosed with pancreatic cancer. Three weeks later, she passed away.

Model Behavior

▼ ▼ ▼

Thanks to more patients and to high school and college friends working and living in New York, I started to meet more people in the city. I had to temper this diversion, though, because a surgeon can have only so active a nightlife, especially a young surgeon consumed with succeeding, and who thought about plastic surgery every waking moment. And New York nightlife, of course, happens late at night, every night. I couldn't stay out late the night before surgery, couldn't drink much, certainly couldn't smoke or do drugs (no deprivation there, since I've never been tempted; why do something that makes you lose control?). On weekends, though, I made an effort to get out. To me, nothing was more exhilarating than sitting around a table and talking with new friends at some downtown spot. These fun, smart, ambitious people were frequently available to do things like that because we were young, unattached, broke, and, well, young. (Some virtues, I know only too well as a plastic surgeon, are attributable simply to the glory of youth—from skin elasticity to the capacity to recover from little sleep.) We were all trying to figure out what would happen to us. Were we among those fortunate ones who would make it in New York? Or would we, at some point down the road, find ourselves tucking our tail between our legs and admitting that we didn't have what it took? I was the straight arrow in a very hip gang that included Nicole Miller (future clothes designer), Patrick McMullen (fashion photographer), Pam Taylor (future marketing maven for the Absolut vodka campaign), and others. Pam said that if she failed, she would go to Europe and be a ski bum. Nicole said she'd go to Tahiti and sell T-shirts. I confessed that I didn't know what

I'd do; I'd already tried going home and it hadn't worked. Back then, if you wanted to have a private practice specializing in cosmetic surgery, you pretty much had to be in New York or Los Angeles. I couldn't just go anywhere and set up a practice. If New York beat me up, then I'd probably return to the Bay Area, or maybe try L.A. Certainly people prized surgically enhanced faces and bodies there.

At parties, whenever Nicole or Pam would introduce me to their friends as "Cap, a plastic surgeon," there would inevitably be a pause or a smile or a laugh or a disbelieving look. It was likely I was the only plastic surgeon at the party. Invariably, a model or young actress, hearing what I did, would sidle up to me and find a way to steal an on-the-spot consult.

"Which are better?" she would quiz me, glassy-eyed, as she pressed her breasts against me. "Silicone or saline?"

I wanted and needed to immerse myself in New York culture, for the camaraderie. But I was a nerd and—thanks to my medical training—a disciplined one. I remember going to a downtown club to see a performance by a young singer named Madonna . . . and having to leave after three songs; I had a browlift scheduled for seven thirty in the morning. There were downtown loft parties with musicians and models and actors, and I would enjoy them—chatting, meeting people—while always surveying the scene as if from above. For me—for most doctors but especially surgeons—a party was a different experience from what it was for lawyers or investment bankers. I stood on the sidelines and watched the counterculture fly by. Still, I enjoyed the parties and nightlife, probably because they represented such a contrast to my day job. Absolute order by day, total recklessness by night—even if my idea of "total recklessness" was, by New York standards, fairly tame.

One Friday night Nicole and I went to The Rave on the Upper West Side. Great music, a lively scene. Coming from work, I stood there in my overly conservative Midwestern suit and a loosened tie, the music pounding, and at one point found myself flanked by two men—one heavily pierced and tattooed, the other in leather. Alcohol was flowing, of course, and patrons were making numerous trips to the bathroom that had nothing to do with relieving themselves. The fashion was outrageous. I remember thinking that, although I'd always tended to see the similarities in people rather than the differences, I was fairly sure there was little overlap between me and the men on either side of me.

A moment later, a group of men in drag walked by . . . and one of them did a double take. I was clearly the reason for his hesitation.

It was one of my patients.

He lived on the straitlaced Upper East Side. He was an investment banker. As straight an arrow as you could find. Two months before, I'd done a nosejob on him.

Had I not seen his eyes, I wouldn't have recognized him. From the way he and his friends were decked out—in heavy makeup, mascara, and tight blouses—he couldn't have expected to be identified. He realized I'd recognized him: His frightened look still burns in my brain. Fortunately for him, I was trained to keep secrets.

I nodded, ever so slightly, hoping to assure him that he needn't worry, at least not about this. His secret was safe.

He returned a tiny, sheepish smile.

My more active social life began to yield some professional benefits. I met a booker at one of the top modeling agencies who referred some of her models to me. At first it was hard for me to believe how many models, including the top ones, underwent surgery. For the most part they wanted liposuction of the hips and the outer thighs, and occasionally breast implants. I would do biopsies of moles and lipomas, too. Back then, liposuction was the most common procedure I did on models; today, it's still lipo, but cheek implants, lip augmentation, and rhinoplasties are common, too. Also, virtually all models have some injections, either Botox or Restylane. And while I did breast augmentations then, it was not yet de rigueur, whereas today, the model who *hasn't* had breast implants is a trailblazer.

Not all models are technically beautiful. Isabella Rossellini, for one, is not a classic beauty, but she photographs well. Most well-known models sport some asymmetry—for instance, Lauren Hutton and that famous gap in her front teeth. (I also thought about Cindy Crawford's mole, and how much I wanted to remove it; I knew it had helped to make her career, but I just didn't get its appeal.) Gisele Bundchen may come closest to technical perfection, but even she has a heaviness in her upper lids.

I did a breast augmentation and multiple small lipos on one struggling model; three weeks later, her booker called to say she'd had her best go-see ever.

Two well-known print models came in, each to have a small bump on her nose removed. After the surgery, their business opportunities expanded; they could now do runway modeling, too.

One particularly homely twenty-year-old came to me for a rhinoplasty, neck lipo, and breast implants, to jump-start a modeling career.

The models were friendly and smarter than you'd think. I thought about asking a couple of them out, but, as a professional, I couldn't do it. It would never work out. My lifestyle and theirs—our hours and our obligations—were incompatible.

One Friday morning I got my biggest model-related job yet—even if the procedure was tiny.

"Francesco Scavullo on the line," said my office manager.

The world-renowned photographer, who had made his name with his signature cover shots for *Cosmopolitan,* was shooting a Danish model for a Victoria's Secret print campaign. She was wearing a string bikini, Francesco was telling me over the phone, and he was bothered by a little smidge of hip fat pinching over the string. Of course I understood what he was saying: Plastic surgeons, fashion photographers, and models see flaws that are imperceptible to others. Scavullo needed to finish the shoot in three days. He and Anna came to my office that afternoon. Right away I could see it would be a relatively easy hip lipo—but what about the bruising?

"I've got to have it done," said Anna. "I need this job. How often do you get to work with Scavullo?"

"Yes, honey," said Scavullo. "You need to have this done."

I couldn't help but be amused. Any guy who saw Anna in this bikini would probably drool; any woman would covet that body, pinch of fat or not. But that's the way it goes. Anna was a victim of the perfectionism of Scavullo, of Victoria's Secret, of the readers of the magazines who saw the ad.

I did the procedure the next morning, a Saturday. We put iced towels on her until Sunday evening, and Scavullo shot on Monday, using concealer to cover what was left of the bruise.

After that, Anna's booking agent, knowing I could help get her clients out of trouble quickly, sent more models my way and even put the word out among former clients, too, that I did professional work.

Working with these new patients, I got to understand, in particular, the poignant predicament of the ex-model. Diane, a well-known former *Sports Illustrated* swimsuit model who had, at thirty-eight, technically finished her modeling career (though she had business ventures on the side), came in to see about a breastlift. She was tall, brunette, and still magnificent, but she'd had a child and she told me she thought her breasts sagged. She was used to their being up and youthful. She was not going to tolerate any aging.

She took off her shirt and bra.

When we measure a breast for "ptosis" (sag), we measure the

distance from the sternal notch—the middle of the chest, between the collarbones—to the nipple. (Of course, much of this can be done simply by looking.) A distance of nineteen to twenty-one centimeters (7½" to 8¼") is considered normal. Anything greater than that is drooping.

Diane had beautifully proportioned breasts. I measured her at twenty-two centimeters—barely sagging.

"It would be easy to do a lift," I said, "and I could even do short-scar surgery. But there would still be a scar on otherwise beautiful breasts that really aren't sagging."

That was not the answer Diane was looking for. "But you would do it," she said.

"I can't see putting a scar on you for such a trivial improvement," I said.

Instead of being happy that she was not a victim of ptosis like other thirty-eight-year-old mothers with relatively sizable breasts, she was disappointed. I would not operate.

She came back a year later, and I measured her again. She had dropped a quarter of a centimer, if that.

She returned a year later. Again, the sag had hardly changed.

It was as if Diane wanted her breasts to sag more. She was in an unfamiliar and uncomfortable place: As an ex-model, she was still gorgeous but she was no longer perfect. And while being ever-so-slightly imperfect would have been more than acceptable to the vast majority of civilian women (or men) out there, Diane seemed to prefer adding scars to her body rather than to accept that time had, if gently, visited her, just as it does everyone else.

Did she go elsewhere to get a breastlift? I don't know.

It used to be that models, both print and runway, were naturally beautiful, with great bone structure and unaltered body shapes.

Starting in the 1980s, this gradually became the exception rather than the norm. The explosion of office-based surgeries, better monitors, and better drugs led to improved cosmetic surgery results. In essence, advances in technology drove aesthetics—and the trend continues today: With injectables, it's now routine for teenagers and women in their early twenties (not to mention older women) to come in for bigger lips, which can be had in ten minutes.

To compete in the hypervisible, hypercompetitive world of modeling, most models now have small to major operations performed. The minor procedures include removal of moles, cauterization of blood vessels, and removal of small lipomas (benign growths of fat); these procedures we do for all models, but now it's trending younger and younger, starting at around age twelve for adolescent models. In the late teenage years, the range of procedures widens to include cheek implants, chin implants, liposuction, and, of course, breast implants. I had a fourteen-year-old model come in, with her mother, wanting breast implants. I told her I didn't do breast augmentation surgery on any girl under sixteen, and frequently I turn down girls for a few years after that. The breast bud is not fully developed then, so I believe it's a mistake to do it that young. (When I turn down the chance to operate on teenage girls, roughly half the time I do it for physical reasons—there's not enough of a defect or the trade-off clearly isn't worth it—and half the time I do it for psychological reasons—because I sense that the girl may not be mature enough to handle it.)

There are more esoteric procedures that models will have, too—removal of ribs, shaving of the jawbone, removal of the buccal fat (fat at the center of our cheeks) to give a more sculpted, haunted look.

Today's plastic surgeons are coming closer and closer to making the face you want. The question is, how far is the subject willing to go? For the model with the potential to make hundreds of thousands, if not millions, of dollars, they'll go very far. Just about every model who comes into my office is determined. A twenty-two-year-old from the Elite agency came in for a breastlift. She was stunning but her breasts were slightly lower than normal, and she needed them lifted if she was going to get runway work. I advised her of the scarring and actually showed her a photograph of a worst-case example. She wasn't fazed at all. She insisted on having the operation. Normally, I wouldn't place a breastlift scar around the areola on a twenty-two-year-old, but that's where she needed it to be, professionally. I also had to modify my technique to ensure that she could breast-feed at a later date.

The range of possibilities in plastic surgery is expanding rapidly each year, and I expect the trend to continue. Soon, we'll truly be able to say that we have "beauty by design."

Katrina, a famous *Vogue* model from Germany, came in at the urging of her agency. As you might expect when a current supermodel comes in for a consult, your first question as a plastic surgeon is, what the hell could this woman possibly need?

You couldn't tell from first glance. Blue eyes, long blond hair, five feet ten, sensational body. She wore jeans, a Nordic sweater, no makeup. Great smile. She was nervous.

Breast implant? Lipo? I wondered. *What on earth could this young woman want?*

"I have a complex," said Katrina. "I have something that's stopping me from getting modeling jobs."

"I find that hard to believe," I said.

"I can do runway but not magazine." She looked down, as if ashamed. "Except if the magazine wants me in a swimsuit."

Then she pulled her hair back.

Her ears were huge and tilted way forward. "I don't know anyone who can fix them," she said, "and my agent said you can."

"It's simple," I said.

It took an hour, using only local.

Removing the bandages afterward, I gently tugged the last strip off and gave her a mirror. Katrina looked and, tentatively, held her hair back. She broke into a big smile. Then she started to cry.

A few days later, the booking agent for the modeling agency called. I thought she wanted to thank me for fixing Katrina's ears.

"I know you've worked on some of our girls, and their bodies are even more incredible," she said. "I'm jealous. I want breast implants, too."

A week after the operation, she called. "You may have to take them out," she said wearily. "I need a baseball bat to keep my husband off."

When I laughed, she said, "I'm serious! Can you at least recommend the best cream for backburns?"

Sometimes, it's almost unbelievable to me how many women want breast implants. Breast augmentation has been one of the hottest things in plastic surgery for a decade, and it's true across social strata. Among beauty role models—actresses, swimsuit and magazine models—its prevalence is huge.

But when the most stunning women in America are getting breast implants, it causes a thought even a cosmetic surgeon must ask: Does everybody really suffer some kind of physical insecurity? Are business demands that great? Have the altered (i.e., enhanced) standards of attractiveness in our culture pressured everyone to feel as if they've got something that needs changing . . . or else they've got nothing?

Yes.

I came to see that everyone, no matter how apparently perfect, has something that bothers him or her. Some hang-up. Something that might be trivial to you but not to them. Jowls, saddlebags, heavy lids, bags under the eyes, bump in the nose, small breasts, big breasts, uneven breasts, male breasts, the list is long. It's true for the not so rich and the very rich, the average-looking and the drop-dead gorgeous. Everyone.

And what those things are five or twenty years from now will almost certainly change. Once, women wanted their hair to look like Veronica Lake's, then Jane Fonda's, then Madonna's, then Jennifer Aniston's. Popular concepts of beauty change and often come from the top down. If Hollywood actresses suddenly decide that flat-chestedness is beautiful, then there likely wouldn't be the same demand among the general public for breast implants.

Then again, the notion of the empowered woman is not a fad but a reflection of sweeping cultural and technological change. Women (first in the West and increasingly everywhere) are more in charge than they have ever been professionally, financially, sexually, physically, psychologically. Most women pay for their own implants, as a gift to themselves. We live more and more in a world in which we're told we can be anyone, where lives are increasingly customized to the individual. Since many women want to have the physique—at least the breasts—of a *Playboy* centerfold, and now they can, and easily, their philosophy is, *Why not?*

While downtown New York and the modeling world were fun, my practice would live or die on my relationships with women uptown (as well as those from other parts of the country and the world). The same was true of any New York cosmetic surgeon. Gradually, I was getting more referrals through patients, and doing more types of procedures. I met people in banking, advertising, and media. I met diplomats and international lawyers—men doing what I'd long ago thought I someday wanted to do. (I had to admit, their lives seemed pretty exciting.) I continued to do the best work I could, hopeful that my patients not only felt transformed by their face-lift, browlift, tummy tuck, or hip liposuction, but also raved about it over lunch with friends.

I got my first taste of international patients. A broadcaster from Hong Kong came in to have me Westernize her eyes, a procedure I'd learned to do at Stanford. "Don't make me look *too* different," she said. "I was beautiful when I was young. Men chased me." Western and Asian eyes, as you might suspect, have different lid anatomies and support structures. The key to an effective "Westernizing" is to take out a little bit of skin from the epicanthic fold of the upper eyelid; this area is nearest to the nose and allows us to change the curve. The other parts of the lid are left alone. The lower lid gets altered only slightly, with fat being removed transconjunctivally—that is, the incision is made inside the lid. I've done far more of those procedures than I have of the reverse—*undoing* Westernized eyes for Asians who want their totally Asian look back. That's much more difficult.

A couple of weeks later, I was dining at a French restaurant when a departing patron, the wife of a wealthy Turkish businessman, caught her heel in a sidewalk grid just outside the restaurant, fell, and broke her nose. After someone rushed inside and hollered, "Is there a doctor?!" I strode outside, examined the woman—the bones had punctured through the skin—and called my nurse to ready my operating room. We got the woman over there. While I sutured her, her husband playfully spun in my OR chair. The next morning, a two-foot cube of Godiva chocolate arrived for my office staff, along with an invitation for me to spend a week on their yacht in the Mediterranean.

A wealthy and intimidating Venezuelan oil magnate came to me to shrink his waistline.

A woman from Australia, whose husband was attached to the United Nations, came for a face-lift. She was so secretive that much of our preliminary contact was through an intermediary, and I finally stressed to her representative that I would not continue until I met the lady in person and could look at her *actual face*. They relented.

One day, an eighty-year-old Italian lady came to the office. She was a recognizable figure: I would regularly see her on Madison Avenue in bright Valentino suits and stilettos. After we talked for a moment, she told me she needed "emergency breast implants."

"Emergency?" I asked.

"I have a date with a hot young man in a week," she said. "Yes, it is an emergency!"

Just then my phone line flashed, and I excused myself to take the call. Before I even had the phone to my ear, I was being pelted by obscenities.

"You son of a bitch! I am going to kill you you son of a bitch! You turned my penis black!"

Who is this lunatic? I wondered.

"Hello?" I said, turning my body away from my consult. Whatever the reason for the invective on the other end, it was unlikely to inspire confidence in the prospective patient now sitting in my office. "Who is this?" I asked, covering the phone with my hand.

"This is Diego, you son of a bitch, you turned my penis black! My testicles are black! You gave me a black penis!"

It was the powerful Venezuelan oil magnate on whom I'd performed waist and hip liposuction two days before.

"May I ask you to hold for one moment?" I said into the phone, then quickly hit the HOLD button. I smiled at the lady in my office and asked her to please excuse me for just one quick little moment. I withdrew to the OR and picked up the line again.

"Now, Diego, take it easy, everything is going to—"

"Take it easy?! Everything is not going to be okay, asshole, especially for you! I have a black penis!"

"Take a breath and—"

"I'm gonna kill you you're dead!"

"Diego?" I could hear him breathing heavily—but pausing long enough for me to speak. "Okay, now, Diego? Everything is going to be fine. You are *not* going to have a black penis. Or black testicles. I promise you. The reason they turned black is that you didn't follow my instructions after the operation. Or really you followed them *too* zealously. Remember I told you to wrap the elastic bandage . . . *not too tight?* How tight did you wrap it?"

His breathing was still heavy, almost wheezing. "Tight," he finally said quietly.

"Very tight, I bet."

There was silence . . . and then what sounded like a deep sigh. "Very tight," he acknowledged.

"I told you not to do that—remember?"

Again, a sigh. "So I'm not going to have a black penis," he said flatly.

"No, you're not. Because you wrapped it too tight, you reduced the returning circulation from the groin. It's backed-up blood. It will be gone within four days."

I hung up with Diego, returned to the eighty-year-old patient in my office, and we scheduled "emergency" breast augmentation for her the following Monday, so she would be ready for her date with the young man the following weekend.

Building a reputation takes time.

About Face,
Skin Deep

▼　▼　▼

I've analyzed the faces of over twenty thousand women. I do it all day, week after week, year after year.

The plastic surgeon sees the face differently from everyone else. Like most people, I look at the eyes and mouth first, then take in the face's coloration. But within milliseconds, I break the face into individual components, then convert them into anatomy. For example, I see a large bump on the nose as if the skin were invisible; I study its cartilage component, its height, width, consistency, boniness.

I find shapes. How does this face depart from da Vinci's description of perfect balance, in which the face divides into three equal parts of forehead, middle third, and lower third? For example, if a patient has a weak chin, I determine if the lowest third of her face is shorter than the upper thirds because of the chin's deficiency. Would a chin implant do the trick? Or should I do an osteotomy—a chin advancement—to increase the length of the lower third of the face, to create the pleasing facial balance the eye craves?

I look for shadows. I look for asymmetries. Is the left side of the lower lip even with the right? To get a sense of the underlying musculature, I again look at the face as if the skin had been removed from it, and it were just muscles underneath. Which muscles are firing? Is the frontalis muscle moving the eyebrows evenly? Are the lip depressor's (depressor anguli) moving the lips evenly?

I look at the face from another angle—does my perception of

the face change more than normally when she turns her head slightly? Now that I'm looking at it from the side, what do I see about the face that I did not see before? Is the jawline straight? Is the nose too big? Are the ears too big? My analysis of the face is multifactorial: I look to see where it is in time, what is in its future, what is its past (scars, sunlight, biopsies). I assess its appearance in light, its anatomy, its genetics (e.g., pale Irish skin heals better, say, than thicker negroid skin).

My antennae are up the moment I walk into my office to meet a new consult. Although I know before I walk into my office what she has called about (even though many patients, particularly women, will change their minds or bring up new issues once we start talking), I like to think that if I didn't have that information, I could still tell right away what the patient is there for, especially if it's for something above the neck. Sir Arthur Conan Doyle, a physician more famously known as the creator of that master deducer Sherlock Holmes, taught a medical school course at the University of Edinburgh in which patients would enter the classroom and his students had to diagnose their illness merely by looking at them.

It's not easy for me to shut off my PSR (Plastic Surgeon's Radar), and I don't believe, among my professional brethren, that I'm alone. A baseball slugger sees a belt-high fastball and thinks, *I can hit it;* a writer overhears a memorable exchange and thinks, *I can write it;* I see a face and think, *I can improve it.* As soon as I see a face—live, in a photograph, in a painting, on a sculpture—I can't help myself (most of the time) from assessing its symphony of features and accents, what is pleasing about it and what is not. Most importantly, as a fixer of faces, I can't help but home in on the things that can be changed, to make it look more appealing, given what I know about medicine, anatomy, aesthetics, perception, and the psychology of seeing.

I was trained to do this, though it's been so long now, perhaps it's become my nature to do it, too. It may seem overly critical and judgmental that I approach faces this way, even cruel. But I don't *volunteer* to people I meet that they should do this or that, or wouldn't it be nice if they had this done or removed some of that? I only share what I know with those who come to me, who ask me to do it, who retain me to do it.

That doesn't stop men and women, but especially women—sometimes dates and romantic interests—from prodding me to tell them, as if it's some kind of game, what's "wrong" with their face, how I would change them, what could be done that would almost certainly make them happier. It's actually an incredibly poignant dynamic, if you think about it: people asking me to tell them what will make their lives better, asking me to guide them closer to some inner beauty by pinpointing what can be done to enhance their outer beauty. As if they didn't have an inkling of it already.

Because I think they already know the answer.

The first thing to "go" in a woman's face, at around age forty-two, are the upper eyelids. (This is not true of every face, of course, and various factors—sun, smoking, genetics, to name three major ones—affect the age at which this happens.) Observers can't help registering this change because when looking at faces, we naturally look first at the eyes. If a woman has a heavy upper lid, then the eye's apertures narrow over time. When I do an eye lift—really, an eyelid lift—it alleviates this narrowing: I remove skin and fat from the upper lid, which opens the eyes once again, and right away the subject appears younger. Roberta, a smart, pretty investment banker I once dated, asked me, after a month of our seeing each other, if I would do an upper-eyelid lift on her. (My PSR was off with her, but now that she asked me about it, I could see what she was talking about. I hesitated to do the operation, but she said she would trust no one else.) Even I was floored to see how beautiful Roberta's blue eyes were, now that the excess skin on her lids had been removed—and I don't mean to say what a high-quality job I had done. But that's just the kind of difference a reversal of that "narrowing" can make.

Facial lines first start to appear in the thirties, then increase and become really visible in the forties—and you know which ones: crow's-feet, glabellar lines (the vertical ones between the eyebrows), and those at the corners of the mouth. The deeper, nasolabial folds, which run from the corners of the mouth to the outer edges of the nostrils, really start to appear more in the late forties and become prominent in the fifties, as do the vertical lines leading to the upper lip. (There's a basic concept any good plastic surgeon knows: Wrinkles form perpendicular to the muscle that's contracting.)

It's also around age forty-five when the neck begins its descent, followed by the jawline. Of course, for those who've spent much time in the sun, all this decay, I'm sorry to say, happens sooner.

You can't talk about aging without talking about skin.

I'd long believed that exfoliation, if done periodically and gently, would not only remove superficial growths but also improve the texture of the skin and improve the homogeneity of pigmentation. I'd been performing dermabrasion with small, custom-made diamond burs, and my patients would come every year to have skin treatments.

But I was still largely ignorant of, and skeptical about, the importance of skin care. Sure, I knew a lot about skin. Surgeons understand skin differently from other physicians because we have extensive experience with its texture, depth, and fat consistency. We understand the course the muscles and nerves take, and how that interacts with skin to create wrinkles. I knew that older, thinner, "atrophic" skin heals better—the wound closes cleaner and the scar is thinner—because a particular type of collagen changes over time. I knew that drier skin heals better than oily skin. That the forehead and nose are naturally more oily, the cheeks and lower lip drier, the upper lip drier still. I knew that patients with larger pores (oilier skin) tended to heal worse. That the skin of the eyelids heals beautifully; the skin in front of the ear, very well; the areola, badly; the skin on the back, terribly. That any skin that covers a joint heals poorly, because it stretches.

But for all this knowledge, I did not come to realize the importance of skin care until several years ago, when a sixty-year-old Frenchwoman with magnificent skin came to my office seeking a necklift. I asked her why her skin was so good. "I go to this lady in Paris," she said, and mentioned the woman's name. (The woman in my office wanted a face-lift because she was quite jowly.)

Six weeks later, another Frenchwoman, sixty-five, came in for a consult, and she, too, had spectacular skin. I asked her why her skin was so good.

"I go to this lady in Paris," she said, and she mentioned the same woman the previous consult had mentioned.

I decided to see for myself. I flew to Paris and tracked down the woman, Odile Lecoin. Her office was routinely filled with magazine editors who swore by her. I asked her about her methods. She had started doing microdermabrasion before anyone else. Twenty years earlier, she told me, she had started facial sanding, using small crystals and an air-blowing machine she'd found in Italy. My microdermabrasion treatments could leave the skin red for a day; Mme. Lecoin's did not. I was mightily impressed with her results and invited her to bring her knowledge of skin care to my office, so that I might expand the skin-care treatments I offered my patients.

She accepted. She worked in my office for five years, incorporating her extensive knowledge of microdermabrasion into the skin-care regimen I had established, and teaching me her secrets. When Mme. Lecoin retired two years ago, I decided to expand our offerings. I developed a technique that, using a new kind of crystal, not only allowed smoothing of the skin, but also the prevention and treatment of skin infections. This was of particular advantage for acne, which is notoriously difficult to treat. Moreover, it did not require the use of antibiotics.

While I was doing this on my own, I was asked by one of the Estée Lauder companies to be a consultant on developing a skin-care line. Why they chose me, I wasn't sure; but I know they'd researched hundreds of plastic surgeons, and I'd heard that some of the Estée Lauder executives had noticed the skin-care results out of my office. At the same time, the CEO of Saks encouraged me to develop a skin-care line. This began a three-year search for me to find chemists to help develop an effective, completely noncosmetic form of skin therapy.

In the meantime, I started collecting, anecdotally and from my own research, thoughts about skin care.

1. It amazes me how many women apply (and overapply) oils and creams to their face—especially women with adult acne or oily skin. If your skin is oily or if you have acne, *DO NOT USE* moisturizer, day creams, or extra oil on that part of your skin. Doing so only makes it worse. I realize that certain soaps and frequent use of soaps dries the skin. But soap comes in different types and strengths, from the extreme of Dial to that of an olive-oil soap. Some of the best skin I've ever seen belongs to women who cleanse with cold water and soap, then apply a mild moisturizer on the dry spots.

2. Ultraviolet light breaks down the collagen bonds in the dermis layer of the skin and can alter the DNA of cells in the base layer. This not only ages the skin but may also give rise to skin cancers such as basal cell cancer, squamous cell

cancer, and melanoma. Skin creams with low SPF factors
(4–20) are ineffective; use a factor greater than 20. But that's
not enough: If you're sweating, the salt degrades SPF factors
after two hours or less. For it to be effective, you need to
reapply it.

3. As I mentioned above, exfoliaton works. Both
   microdermabrasion—a spraying of fine crystals at the skin
   to loosen dead tissue—and its forebear, dermabrasion, work.
   They make your skin smoother and help to remove brown
   spots. Everyone should incorporate them into their regimen.
   How frequently you need it depends on your skin. If you
   have lots of little bumps and growths on your skin or your
   skin is blotchy, you need more frequent treatments. If you're
   younger and your skin is smoother, you need fewer
   treatments.

4. To treat wrinkles, brown spots, and blotchy skin, get the
   real thing—not a cosmetic but something that has medicine
   in it to correct hyperpigmentation. The state-of-the-art skin
   lightener is a drug called hydroquinone. The maximum
   strength allowed for over-the-counter medicines is 2 percent.
   In my office, I custom-make a skin lightener with 5 percent
   hydroquinone and add a small amount of cortisone to
   increase its ability to penetrate the skin. Because of the
   higher percentage of hydroquinone, this custom blend can
   only be distributed by my office, since a prescription is
   required. It's because of my frustration with the limitations
   of cosmetics that I'd worked to develop my own skin-care
   line, which includes a set of proteins that allows medicines
   to penetrate the skin better, to make skin pigment more
   homogeneous, and to plump up the lips.

   There have been reports that hydroquinone is possibly
   carcinogenic. When I looked into these reports, I saw that
   they were few, and that the mice were bathed for weeks in

hydroquinone. So I'm skeptical of hydroquinone's potential for causing cancer. Nonetheless, I will incorporate some newer proteins into my skin-care line that have the same effect as hydroquinone but with no potential carcinogenic issues.

5. Lots of money is spent on products that claim they can eliminate or reduce stretch marks. I've never seen them work. I doubt they *could* ever work because stretch marks are caused by a loss of elastin proteins in the thickness of the dermis. To work, then, these products would have to penetrate the skin deeply so that they could change the skin's actual protein composition. And if that were the case, these products would be required to undergo testing by the Food and Drug Administration; if they passed those tests, they would be prescription medicines.

Most skin-care products don't work. Some do, to an extent. Moisturizers form a thin barrier of oil that prevents one's own moisture from evaporating, thus leaving the skin plump. Glycolic acids and peels can change the natural collagen and make it more "organized" in its appearance—that is, tighten the skin. For the most part, though, skin-care products are just cosmetics that mask what's actually going on in the skin. A cosmetic does not actually protect or change the skin.

As I became more aware of my patients' skin conditions and desires, after working with multiple chemists, and after spending years doing research at Cornell and New York University, I was ready to start my own skin-care line, which would offer products that were *medicinal,* and which would make no exaggerated claims. I call my products anticosmetics. Every cream or lotion I develop must have medicinal qualities, must have a delivery system that enables deep penetration, and must do so without irritating the skin or reducing the skin's natural barrier to infection. I demanded from my chemists that we avoid the stock lotions that are the basis for almost all the cosmetics currently on the market. Every ingredient would have a function. All fragrances and colorations would be removed. And unlike other products, mine would include pharmaceutically pure substances whenever possible. These substances would probably cost more, but they would be unique and effective.

Despite the time I spent researching and developing a skin-care line, I kept my focus on plastic surgery. My sense of medical discipline made me follow the same pre-op routine with every procedure. The routines were drilled into me in medical school and during my residencies, and they could not be circumvented. I reviewed a checklist to minimize the chance that something could go wrong, then reviewed a checklist for how to handle those moments if something did go wrong. Before the operation, my staff and I together went over everything. Then, even though we'd checked everything once, when the patient was wheeled in for surgery, we checked it all again.

The monitors.

The oxygen tanks.

Were all the necessary drugs and medications within arm's reach?

If the power failed, did everyone know what to do?

If the patient went into cardiac arrest, did everyone know what to do?

It was like a fire drill, or a pilot going through his sequence. And just as the pilot had a ground crew to check instruments for him preflight, when he got to the plane, it was up to him to check everything again.

As to the particular procedure, I reviewed it in the days leading up to, then again right before, the operation.

My OR environment had its unbreakable rules, too. No piped-in music. No chitchat. No food or drink. No pictures on the wall. No singing. No phone calls.

My office was in a perfect spot, on Park and Sixty-fifth. I played classical music in the waiting room. Across the street was Daniel, the popular French restaurant. Central Park was blocks away. This was the alpha and omega of a Park Avenue practice. I had a Westchester practice, too. Good results were all I wanted. Being in the OR—gowned, gloved, in my mask, instruments ready, operating, transforming—became my sanctuary, my temple.

I was in a zone.

Women of the World
▼ ▼ ▼

The more my practice grew, and the more diverse my clientele became, the more I was able to say, from my own fund of experiences, that people of different ethnicities, nationalities, and races had particular tendencies. Plastic surgery had come a long way and expanded into every one of these different groups. It became clear that now everyone, regardless of background, had something that bothered him or her. For some, it was groupthink; for others, physical expediency.

For example, when Scandinavian women come in for breast surgery, many more ask for reductions than augmentations. Fortunately for them, the genetics of their skin make them heal the best of pretty much any ethnic or racial group; the scars are finer, flatter, smoother.

Italians often come in for rhinoplasties, to reduce and straighten that famous "Roman nose." Once, at a medical conference, I was presenting photographs of some large noses I'd operated on. A doctor from Turin stood. "I bet I've worked on bigger ones," he boasted, holding up photos of his own nasal subjects. (He was right.) Italian women also love flat bottoms. Southern Italians have naturally oily, olive skin that heals poorly, yielding wider scars and more pigment around the scars than northern-European skin. The surgeon must be more aware of where he puts his incisions.

Because Frenchwomen smoke a lot, they tend not to heal well. They like face-lifts but they're insistent that the look be natural, subtle; in twenty years, I've never had a Frenchwoman (or one from Madrid) who wanted a face-lift that looked even remotely pulled. They like big lips. For some reason I can't explain, Parisian women, contrary to expectation, rarely use makeup well—or maybe, to my eye, they wear too much. They're as stylish as any group of women in the world and understand the use of color for their face. However, their application of eyelid makeup and lipstick can be excessive. (I would not venture this opinion if I were the only plastic surgeon who has noted it.)

Thanks to the liberal French medical system, women and men tend to use far more injectables—vitamins and misotherapy—to treat wrinkles than elsewhere in Europe and the United States. Unfortunately, there is much mystery about what's in some of these injectables. Sometimes they're mixed with silicone or other foreign materials, which frequently leads to reactions and infections. (In my experience, only South Americans and Mexicans get infected more than the French; they, too, are often injected with silicone contaminated with bacteria.) These infections can be nasty. Because silicone is a foreign material, it rarely clears from the system with just antibiotics, and the infection persists until the material is surgically removed.

Spanish women—perhaps the most elegant international group I deal with—come in for lipos, face-lifts, lip augmentations, and pretty much everything else, and they come back for multiple procedures. I've tended to develop a rapport with them, perhaps because my first-ever Spanish patient—a member of the royal family—turned out so well (she was thrilled with the result) that I received numerous referrals. Around Christmastime, I frequently receive phone calls from Málaga, Seville, or Madrid saying, "Cap, how are you? . . . May I come in January for a quick fix?"

I have not developed such a rapport with German women. They break appointments, frequently change their mind about what operation they want done, and can be fairly demanding. Like Scandinavian women, they also get lots of breast reductions. They like liposuction, particularly for the outer leg.

Hispanic women come for lipo on every body part but the rear, which they prefer to look like Jennifer Lopez's. (In fact, sometimes they ask for buttock implants or fat grafts to the buttocks.)

Brazilians don't care so much about scarring, which can in their case be hard to disguise because of their generally dark pigmentation, given the large Indian influence in their genetic pool. Dr. Ivo Pitanguy made Brazil the center of cosmetic surgery in the 1970s by getting Brazilian surgeons to publish in Western medical journals and by masterfully marketing himself. Because of this, and because Brazilians love the outdoors and curvy bodies, they have an extraordinary amount of breast augmentation. Billboards on freeways advertise breast implants. This is a somewhat recent development; the Brazilian ideal—"the girl from Ipanema"—used to be svelte, almost flat-chested. Girls in Brazil get breast implants way too young, younger even than American girls (though ours are catching up).

Argentinians—not as body-conscious as Brazilians, and on average a little heavier—mostly come in for facial work. Their skin quality is mostly of northern Italian and European background, so they heal better than Brazilians.

Venezuelan women are beautiful and showy. For the Miss Venezuela beauty pageant, contestants who've had plastic surgery don't merely refrain from hiding it; they flaunt it. They like large breasts, slim hips, and full lips. They do not like big rears.

Colombians do like big rears. In one unfortunate instance, a lawyer from Bogotá wanted her buttocks built up, so she injected herself with filler, which caused an infection. When she came to see me about it, she had two infected cheeks, each with a bright red dimple. I told her she had two choices: take antibiotics and hope that it killed the infection (unlikely) or have all the subcutaneous tissue cut out of her buttocks. Not surprisingly, she opted first to try the antibiotics. Within a month, fortunately, they worked.

For a small country, Peru is quite chic. I have worked on both the more Indian-inflected Peruvians and the more European ones (who tend to come to me when they're younger). Peruvians have more facial work than body work. They are unusually worldly, maybe more so than my clients from any other country in South America. They can tell me what plastic surgeons are doing in London, Paris, and Madrid.

Asian women consider scarring a horrible stigma. A scar is "impure" and damages their chances of marrying. A Chinese flight attendant, accompanied by the managing director of her airline, came to see me for a consultation. She had been burned in a crash in China, and had a two-by-three-inch scar on her forearm. In the grand scheme, the burn was hardly huge, and many people would have adapted psychologically. Not her. And not him. He spoke respectfully about his employee. "Dr. Lesesne," he explained to me "in our culture a scar like this is devastating. To remove it is extremely important not only to our employee but to our company."

Korean women want three procedures more than any others, one of which I won't do. Because Koreans have a genetic disposition to bowleggedness, many wish to reduce the outer bowing of the lower leg (the tibia and fibula bones), and some women request that the legs be broken and then set straighter. I know there are surgeons in Korea who will do this. I won't. There's a high chance of complication and a mal-union of the bones. If the leg doesn't heal right, they may have trouble walking.

Koreans also have square mandibles, or lower jaws, and want the jaw narrowed. This requires making an incision inside the mouth, using a bur or sanding tool to shave off part of the jaw, then cutting it in the back and resetting it. Koreans also want to reduce the width of their cheeks, which also requires sanding down bone (the maxilla and zygoma, the two bones that make up the cheek). These procedures I do.

Many Japanese women like to have their faces appear more oval; they never ask for cheek or chin implants, which make the face look angular. Nor do Japanese women ask for upper-lip augmentation; the geisha, a still-prominent beauty icon, paints her mouth so that the lower lip looks full but the upper lip thin.

Asian women also often want nasal augmentation, which entails adding cartilage to build up the depressed bridge of a relatively flat nose. In many places in Asia, doctors will do something we don't do nearly as much here—augment the nose with a silicone block. Since it's impossible to completely sterilize the nasal passages during surgery, bacteria can get on the silicone and the body can't clear it, which can lead to a long-term infection. The body's natural response to a chronic infection is to extrude, or push out, the material to the surface. Several Asian women have come to the office with nasal implants so infected, they were starting to poke through the skin.

The Chinese women I see tend to be taller than the Japanese and Korean women, not as genetically isolated, and seem more willing to change their bodies than the Japanese, in particular (though Korean-American women are moving more in that direction, too). Chinese women are more likely than other Asians to want their eyes Westernized. They like breast implants. At least once a year I'll go to Hong Kong to do consults (though most of my native Asian patients I'll see when I consult in Los Angeles). In Hong Kong, many of the consults come in with their boyfriends, having expressed interest in only face and nose work. But as soon as they're in the hotel room, the women—clearly at the urging of their boyfriends—ask for breast implants, too. A common refrain is "My *tai tai*"—their phrase for a wealthy and Westernized Hong Kong man—"thinks I'm too flat."

▼

What are some of the regional plastic surgery preferences of Americans?

Few patients want overly pulled face-lifts, but occasionally I get someone who requests it—and invariably she is from either New York or L.A.

Midwesterners and New Englanders are the most reserved personally and are emphatic that the work be undetectable. When they come in for rhinoplasties, they rarely want me to do anything to the tip. Midwesterners just want the bump removed, thank you. I've noticed that Midwesterners tend to influence their family: If a woman comes in and she's happy with the results, soon enough her sister will come in, too. Midwesterners also tend to get lots of lipo, and more breast reductions than women from other regions. (Because of the long, harsh winters, they tend not to exercise as much as those in other parts of the country.)

Northeastern women want breast implants but (generally) not big ones. When they have nosejobs, they'll want more tip work.

Because they are so diverse, it's hard to generalize about Californians. Southern Californians typically seek body sculpting, breast implants, and injectables, especially to the lips. These injectables can be fat grafts, collagen, Restylane, or the more permanent Radiesse. Although the plastic surgery aesthetic in Southern California, particularly around Los Angeles, tends to be overt, the patients who come to me from that region are looking for subtlety (or else they'd just find someone in their own backyard).

Texans are attractive and well put-together. They want face-lifts, face-lifts, face-lifts. Texans do not have breast reductions. In all my years of practice, I have yet to do one on a Texan.

Southerners (excluding Floridians) show up at my office well-dressed, perfectly made up, and with their hair almost always neatly pulled back. They are unfailingly polite. They are trim—never skinny, and never, ever, ultrathin. Southerners want the same procedures everyone else wants, but they are extremely concerned about scars; as common as cosmetic surgery is becoming down there, they want to be discreet about it.

There are two types of Florida women: those indigenous to the state, and the transplanted New Yorkers, who are older and often retired. The retirees want face-lifts and other facial surgery, and usually it's not their first visit. No matter how fastidious a young, native Floridian has been about her skin care, she has sun damage and wants facial work. The younger ones, especially in South Florida, are very aware of their bodies and want breast implants, usually very big ones. One woman from Miami came in wanting implants bigger than I would have recommended for her frame. But after many phone calls Tara wore me down and finally I acquiesced. "Okay," I said. "If that's what you really want, I'll put in four hundred seventy-five cc's instead of two-fifty, but please don't come back to me complaining that they're too big." I did the operation in October; she failed to show up for her follow-up visit.

In February, the phone rang. It was Tara.

"Dr. Lesesne, I was in a terrible Rollerblading accident in South Beach," she said. "I went flying right in front of all the cafés, and I have terrible injuries to my skin, my knees, my arms." I told her I was sorry to hear that and was just waiting for her to blame it all on the size of her breasts.

"And I would have broken my ribs, too," she said, "if not for those big, wonderful breasts!"

Sometimes, the patient knows better than the doctor what's right for her.

Competition

▼ ▼ ▼

I felt fortunate to have a thriving plastic surgery practice on Park Avenue. But I knew I was only as good as my last result. I knew that if I was ever anything but "on," I'd be in trouble. I knew that I had to be aware of what my colleagues were doing, yet not lose focus on my own work.

Because as much as I wanted to succeed, lots of people out there did *not* want that.

The perception is that the "fraternity" of plastic surgeons, especially those who cater to a certain clientele and who themselves live richly—especially those of the Park Avenue variety—is hardly a fraternity at all, and that backstabbing is rampant.

For the most part, that's not true—though at times it can be.

It takes immense training and sacrifice to make it here. The Gold Coast—Park, from Sixty-fourth Street to Seventy-second Street—is home to some of the most renowned plastic surgeons in the world. While once Brazil was *the* destination for top-of-the-line cosmetic surgery, New York has surpassed it, with Los Angeles, Miami, and Dallas not far behind.

Plastic surgeons, especially those along the Gold Coast, are my rivals, but they're my colleagues, too. Sometimes we exchange information or opinions. I've shared new techniques with others. A colleague called to ask if, when doing a necklift, I dissect under the platysma muscle. "Dissect *under*?" I said. "I go *five inches* under." He asked me how, and if it was safe, and I advised him that he should make sure, when cutting, to turn his scissors vertically, not horizontally.

I've had colleagues generously share with me. Richard Swift, an excellent plastic surgeon, told me about a technique he'd discovered when doing a canthopexy (tightening of the lower lid) that was simpler and yielded better results than what I'd been doing, a method that also had valuable implications for reconstructive work.

As with any hypercompetitive pursuit, then, you stay on top by working hard but also by sharing with those around you who can help.

You also stay on top—or keep from getting bounced off—by assuming that your competitors every now and then crave nothing more than a little schadenfreude—that is, pleasure over your failure.

A Park Avenue address gives you enormous cachet, so of course the jockeying to plant your stake there is ferocious. You want to be the man, but so does everyone else. To begin with, not every plastic surgeon in the city has a private practice; less than half do. It's staggeringly expensive to set one up and maintain it, easily more than $300,000 a year. Then your facility had better be accredited, and highly, by one of the three most important organizations—the Joint Commission on Hospital Accreditation (JCOH), the American Association of Ambulatory Facilities (AAA), and the American Association for Accreditation of Ambulatory Surgical Facilities (AAAA). They make sure your OR is set up for quality control, safety, and fire hazards, meaning you've got to implement policies and procedures and buy all kinds of equipment: crash carts, backup power supply, backup water supply, etc. My office is accredited by the JCOH—in my opinion, the most rigorous of the three ranking bodies.

Some New York plastic surgeons work at a hospital, and that's it. Some are in private practice, but not on Park.

The ones on Park are at once the most esteemed and reviled.

So it's no wonder that many "colleagues" gossip or even actively plot to bring each other down.

One prominent, highly skilled colleague was rumored to have attempted suicide. He did not. He recovered from the fallout of the rumor to have his practice thrive, deservedly, once more.

Another plastic surgeon was rumored to be a cross-dresser. Also not true.

Recently, the New York grapevine produced this bit of juicy gossip: One of my fellow plastic surgeons, and a role model of mine, had AIDS.

His practice took a hit. A big one.

The rumor, it turned out, was untrue. It was started by a "colleague," a surgeon who'd been envious for years of his target's success.

Innuendo can put you out of commission a long time. It can destroy reputations, careers, relationships. A starry-eyed patient who'd had romantic designs on her plastic surgeon circulated so many rumors about his sexual exploits—that he had slept with patients, that he was with multiple women at once—that his girlfriend finally broke up with him. But it was all fabricated. It was unclear whether the girlfriend left because she believed the charges, or because she hated that he was such an easy target for salacious rumors.

Another colleague tried to drive several competitors, including me, out of town, by exploiting a faulty complaint system. Dr. Jack (we'll call him) repeatedly called New York State's Office of Professional Medical Conduct with bogus or inflated claims about surgeries that other plastic surgeons had done. (New York's OPMC is the only place in the country where, amazingly, you can make charges against a doctor *anonymously*.)

Dr. X shouldn't have put in a breast implant on Patient A because she had a tram flap with compromised blood supply.

Dr. Lesesne shouldn't have operated on Patient B because she had cancer.

In the latter case, the patient had such advanced cancer of the chest wall (which I knew about; that's *why* I was performing surgery), it had eroded through her skin so that her rib was exposed. What I did not realize was that underneath the scabs were dead tissue and maggots. I cleaned the wound and did an extensive "debridement" (removing dead tissue)—but that left her lung partially exposed. I took tissue from her back (the area over the latissimus muscle), tunneled it underneath her arm, and placed it on the front part of her chest, to provide an airtight closure.

The OPMC may or may not investigate a charge—but if it does, and word gets around, it's certainly not *good* news for your practice, even if you're exonerated. When I got wind that Dr. Jack was regularly making charges against other surgeons and me, I called his bluff; I phoned the OPMC myself.

"I would like you guys to investigate me," I said.

I could hear the man turn the phone away and call out to his officemate, "Hey, Barry! We got a doc who *wants* to be investigated!"

Not only was I vindicated, it prompted me to defend other innocent surgeons targeted by the OPMC. That's not to suggest that I will defend a surgeon who I believe may hurt people in the future; unlike the popular belief that doctors protect other doctors, good surgeons subsidize bad surgeons by having to pay inflated insurance premiums. More important, though, I, like most surgeons, care about patients and our fellow man and want to protect and help them.

Bad-mouthing another surgeon reflects as badly on the bad-mouther and will come back to haunt him. If there's a highly flawed surgical outcome walking around that he knows a colleague is responsible for, he shouldn't talk because he doesn't know all the facts. It might happen to him. If patients talk to you about other surgeons (as they do), then they'll surely talk to other surgeons about you, too. Give them only good things to say.

Where once the plastic surgeons' fraternity (if you will) valued the presentation of scientific papers that forwarded ideas, techniques, and methodologies, now the overriding value, and one "shared" with far less fraternal spirit, is the ability to market yourself. (I realize this is a common gripe made across many professions.) Big-time surgeons in New York, Dallas, and L.A. send out promotional videos to patients and print and TV outlets. A recent consult told me she had just gotten such a video from one of the surgeons featured on the reality TV show *Extreme Makeover*. Popular surgeons have—I kid you not—*major ad budgets*. Some send press kits to magazine editors. "Name recognition" becomes the predominant criterion for choosing a surgeon. Recently, I scrubbed with a young plastic surgeon at Manhattan Eye, Ear & Throat Hospital. During the breast implant operation, the second question he asked me was "Who's your PR agent?"

"I don't have one," I said.

He stared at me as if I had a disease. "Are you stupid?"

The new breed of plastic surgeon thinks that media exposure— not word of mouth, not quality of work, not trust—drives your career.

Is it really necessary for a *doctor* to have a publicist? Maybe. I hope not. I always thought that if I worked hard, stayed current, and contributed to my profession, people would find me. But such a route is becoming as anachronistic as my father's house-call-making doctor.

In fact, it feels as if every year I have fewer real colleagues, and more competitors—and that's not paranoia talking, but the reality of a new age. When I started, only board-certified plastic surgeons were allowed to do cosmetic surgery. Now, certain major cosmetic procedures (face-lifts and some large liposuctions) are performed by anyone—dermatologists; ear, nose, and throat (ENT) surgeons; dentists; oral surgeons; obstetricians; and general surgeons. Different boards, with different requirements, oversee these practitioners. None of them, in my opinion, guarantee the rigor of a legitimate plastic surgery training program. So while demand for plastic surgery has gone way up, so has supply, and the people providing the new expertise are not necessarily experts. (Some are good at what they do, some aren't.)

That's not to say that as individuals we don't respect and even like each other. I enjoy seeing some of my peers with whom I trained at New York Hospital. I'll run into surgeons I know at conferences and occasionally social functions. But I tend not to socialize with them, and that reticence is not uncommon. In fact, at times I think we avoid each other's company. It's just the nature of the competition. Plastic surgeons tend to be loners. (A chicken/egg question: Do loners become plastic surgeons? Or does the training and regimen of plastic surgery, and the sometimes constant barrage of patient demands, cause us to retreat into ourselves?)

I enjoy helping younger surgeons, and exchanging ideas with older ones, too, particularly discussing how we deal with complicated cases. There's patient-sharing, too: We'll send prospective consults to each other for second opinions. Or we'll help in other ways. A younger colleague performed a tummy tuck and the patient developed a bad scar, possibly from clotting or a dressing that was wrapped too tightly. The doctor said it was correctable, but the patient quickly turned hostile and threatened to sue. I called the doctor, an acquaintance, to see if I could help. He sent me the chart. He asked my opinion on how he'd done the surgery technically. He hadn't done anything actionable. He put my name in the chart. Even though the problem was fixable, the patient followed through with his threat to sue. When he saw my name on the doctor's chart, he sued me, too.

We also compete against *and* along with each other, at the

same time—at least implicitly, city versus city. While the majority of patients obviously use their local plastic surgeons, a large portion of our clientele is extremely wealthy, jets around easily, and seeks the best that money can buy. This means that lots of our patients come from other cities—or, alternatively, New York patients can migrate elsewhere. New York surgeons, for instance, are in constant battle with surgeons from L.A., Dallas, and Miami. Recently, the Dallas group has published more papers and courts and gets more media attention. On the other hand, a hefty portion of their local client base (Fort Worth, in particular) continues to fly to New York for cosmetic procedures rather than use the plastic surgeons twenty miles away in Dallas. L.A. doctors, as a group, are known for their body sculpting, as are Brazil's surgeons. Dallas does lots of noses and breast implants. For a while, Kansas City had perhaps the best thighplasty person. There's natural and constant competition for patients, and each city's reputation can shift, too.

Other professional arrows, ones not aimed at us explicitly, can also wound us. "Brilliantly innovative surgeon," for example. Sounds like a positive thing, yes? It is—except when the brilliantly innovative surgeon is less cautious than he ought to be.

First, let's take a *genuine* trailblazer. In the 1980s, Dr. Carl Hartrampf, an unassuming giant in our field, pioneered using the abdominal muscle, along with its overlying skin and fat, to reconstruct the breast, postmastectomy. This provided breasts—not implants—that were natural feeling and looking.

Then there are the envelope pushers who are not quite as thoughtful as Dr. Hartrampf; in fact, they promote procedures that ultimately fail. In the early nineties, several surgeons experimented with an "advanced" technique for breast reconstruction:

They harvested the latissimus (back) muscle, tunneled through the skin of the armpit, and inserted the muscle underneath the skin on the chest. The muscle was then folded to make a new breast mound. Novel idea—we're always looking for new sources of tissue—except for one problem: When not being flexed, the latissimus muscle atrophies in sixteen to twenty months. No one knew that initially. The first papers published about the procedure talked up its benefits, reporting no problems.

Two years later, women who'd undergone the revolutionary process suffered loss of breast volume. The muscle shrank and another reconstruction had to be done.

Another example: Other "innovators," looking to give the neck more definition, ran silicone threads underneath the neck. It looked great for the first couple of months. Then it eroded through the skin and the patient felt as if she were being choked.

Or soybean implants. This was a potentially good idea because we were looking for a breast implant filler that was more radiolucent (easily read) for mammographies than saline. Soybean implants were developed in Switzerland and initially manufactured and marketed only in Europe. Unfortunately, the soybean implants experienced some leakage, and when the soybean oil came into contact with fat, it soponified—that is, it broke down the fat in the breast, creating a liquid gel of degraded fat that looked like pus. Since almost all implants have a risk of leakage, they all had to be removed, for fear that any mishap could lead to cancer. Women who'd had soybean breast implants experienced pain, and their breasts were deformed so that they were neither round nor soft.

No innovations would happen in medicine and science without lots of mistakes and wrong paths being taken. Still, I prefer to wait at least a year before I'm willing to try someone's new technique, no matter how promising—especially because no medical board has to ratify a new procedure.

(One surgeon on the Upper East Side may have considered himself an innovator or may just have been misguided. A patient wanted buttock implants. The surgeon decided, inexplicably, to place breast implants in her rear. After she healed, she had . . . well, breast implants in her rear. Whereas buttock, calf, and cheek implants are made of solid silicone, breast implants are hollow and have a fill of either saline or silicone gel. Thus, the feel of a breast implant differs substantially from a buttock implant. The patient was unhappy with the result and went to another doctor. In the exam room during the pre-op visit, the patient—not a native English speaker—told the nurse that she was there to have breast implants removed. The nurse told her, "Take off everything above the waist." The woman replied, "Why?")

Another nasty bit of business about our profession casts dark shadows on many of us—the one that has to do with our motives.

Why does a man become a plastic surgeon in the first place?

The first answer is that he believes in helping people. But when a plastic surgeon becomes more specialized in cosmetic surgery, it means that the vast majority of his waking life will now be spent with women. Surgeons are, by and large, a rather testosterone-charged group of men, and it surprises me that some of my colleagues refer to women in the coarsest terms. Their motivations to enter cosmetic surgery are different from most of ours. Sometimes I think that they simply dislike women, and their professional pursuit allows them the chance to mold and control them.

Did they go into cosmetic surgery with this agenda? Or did it develop after they began working so extensively with women? I don't know. Another chicken/egg question.

▼

A sales representative for a new laser manufacturer visited the office. Meetings like this are common for doctors—reps from pharmaceutical companies and medical technology companies promoting their products. One manufacturer after another had been boasting about how their laser was an improvement over previous versions—good for skin care and removing lines—but especially their miraculous new capability of removing scars.

I told the rep I was frankly amazed that scars could be removed since they're the full thickness of the skin. "I have a rowing scar on my forearm," I said, rolling up my sleeves. "Let's get rid of it."

His eyes widened.

"You set the parameters on the machine," I instructed him.

Nervously, he did.

Not only did the laser burn me, it discolored my arm. I was sore for six weeks. My scar remains, and to this day, lasers don't work well on scars.

To understand better what my patients experience—that is, to be a better doctor—I did everything possible to feel what they went through. When Botox came into fashion, I tried it on myself, injecting it into my forehead. (It hurts.) I lipoed my neck. (Painless, but I felt lumps of dried blood underneath the skin, which took a month to disappear.) I am not a salesman, looking to push new techniques and technologies and medications on my patients just because someone out there says it's the new next best thing. And I would not be one of those doctors who upgrades his knowledge simply by taking a weekend crash course at a Las Vegas convention center.

Do I compete against the best plastic surgeons in the world, especially when it comes to faces and necks? Absolutely. That sounds arrogant, I know. But I have to think that way; I have to believe that's true. Many other surgeons are tremendously talented, some a few doors down from me, some on Rodeo Drive in Beverly Hills, or Harley Street in London, or The Peak in Hong Kong, or Ipanema in Rio de Janeiro, or in Dallas or in Miami or in smaller cities. We see the same patients and I compare my results to what I see from them in my office.

To compete, you must be relentless.

Aging Beauties,
Rediscovered Youth

▼ ▼ ▼

Caroline, a forty-two-year-old Texan, was spunky and attractive: black leather Louboutin boots, leather skirt, light blue cashmere sweater, an ornately knotted Hermès scarf, Gucci sunglasses pushing back her light brown hair. She had brown eyes and rosy cheeks and an infectious smile—but these days she wasn't so crazy about her smile, or her eyes, which is why she'd come to me. As a recent divorcée, she'd been too long out of the dating and mating game and had stopped exercising. She was at that stage of life when the cumulative effects of gravity manifest on a woman's face. The upper eyelids go first with excess heavy skin. The jawline develops fat deposits and excess skin. The neck becomes loose. The mouth turns down. Caroline wanted her looks back so she could recapture companionship, sex, and a place in the social pecking order she craved as a middle-aged divorcée. That's not to say all these good things happen the instant you wake from a face-lift, or an eye lift and a lip plumping. But Caroline was ready to start the transformation.

During the consultation in my office, I agreed that we could do something about the excess fat in her lids, and that her lips, while shaped perfectly, were small. For Caroline, a fat graft would not only make her lips fuller and sensual, but fill out the small vertical lines—called *rhytides* ("lines," in Latin)—leading to the lips where lipstick smudges and bleeds. An eyelid lift, where I cut excess fat out of the upper lid, would open the aperture of her eyes and give her a youthful alertness. (You can get *too* carried away with this procedure, though: For those with naturally heavy upper lids—Julie Christie and Faye Dunaway come to mind—taking out lots of skin can ravage natural, sultry beauty.)

Given Caroline's lively face and her effervescent personality, I was sure she'd look better, younger by three or four years. She smiled a beautiful smile—fine cracks and all—big enough to light up San Antonio's Riverwalk at night.

Three weeks after the consult, Caroline showed up for her surgery at eight, nervous but excited. In the exam room, Caroline got ready—changed into a gown, took off her jewelry. I reviewed the operation with her, as I do with all my patients, then I wheeled her into my OR.

Just before my longtime anesthesiologist, Lisa, gave Caroline propofol to usher her into a "twilight" state (sleeping lightly but arousable), Caroline lay there, looking up at me, as I scrubbed.

"Ready?" I asked.

She nodded, and her right arm emerged from under the sheet. At first I thought she wanted to hold my hand. Lots of patients want that comfort and assurance right before they go under. *Doctor, tell me I won't die. . . . You know what you're doing, right? . . . I'm going to look better when it's over, right? . . . I'll wake up in less than two hours, right?* In fact, in the fourteen years that Lisa and I have been working together, she and I have devised our own light anesthesia cocktail partly because so many women from one particular patient cluster—breast augmentation candidates in their late thirties with young children—exhibit a mortal fear of being put under.

If anything happens to me, what will happen to the children?
Nothing's going to happen, I reassure them—
I have to get back to my kids. . . .

So I started doing those breastlifts and implantations, and others, with an even lighter anesthesia where, ninety seconds after the drip is turned off, the patient is close to fully awake. And can get back to the kids right away. And still have better breasts than she's had since freshman year of college.

Caroline held out her hand—but it wasn't hand-holding assurance she wanted. She was clutching an envelope, which she now thrust toward me. The nurse took it and put it in my scrub pocket.

"Open it *after* the surgery," Caroline said in her soft, south Texas lilt. "Okay?"

I nodded. "Okay."

The whole operation was over in fifty minutes.

In the recovery room, I waited for Caroline to awaken. I looked at her in profile. She was a pretty girl resting peacefully, eyes shut. Her eyes would soon open, and she would begin to talk—as most patients do. Within five minutes, she would be fully alert.

Then I remembered the envelope she'd given me before surgery. I pulled it out of my pocket. In it, on expensive, cream-colored stationery with an embossed red border, was a handwritten note:

Will you have dinner with me next Thursday?

Time.

It works on all of us, constantly, but sometimes it appears as if it's more unfair to some. Too many women who've reached "that certain age" are made to feel undervalued, even invisible, by society, particularly by men. (This is probably more true in our youth-obsessed country than in others.) Not only is it unfortunate for those women who feel underappreciated because of their age, but also as a society we are sacrificing the considerable contributions that these women have to offer.

Fortunately, however, because of the many positive developments for women over the last ten to twenty years, more "women of a certain age" than ever are expressing optimism about the sec-

ond half of their life; this period needn't be characterized by di-
minishment but by opportunity, self-expression, and freedom.
After divorce or tragedy, some women—as with any of us—
retreat. It's natural and important to go through grieving. But
when that's done (or at least manageable), many women resolve to
live life to the fullest, often with an unprecedented determination
and forthrightness. And while the majority of divorcées and widows I operate on are quite interested to meet a man, it's not always
why they've come to me. Lainie, sixty, had been widowed the previous year. I worked with her daughter, Lynnette, a gentle nurse at
one of the New York hospitals where I'm an attending surgeon.
One day Lynnette approached me shyly, to ask if her mother
could come see me.

Any notion that this sweet, reticent young nurse had inherited
her demeanor from her mother was gone soon after Lainie entered
my office, sat down, and answered my question about what she
wanted.

"Well, I want more than one procedure," she said, reasonably
enough, then paused. It was a pause I've experienced hundreds,
even thousands, of times in my career; the moment when a patient
is finally able to say—to this stranger, this man—what she thinks is
most wrong with her. Not an easy moment for anyone.

That's all right, you just tell me what you had in mind—

"I want my forehead lifted," she said, "my upper eyes, my
lower eyes, my nose, my lips, my face, my neck, my arms, my
breasts, my hips, my outer legs, my inner legs, and my ankles."

She took a breath and smiled. "And my stomach."

I waited a moment, to see if more was coming, though she'd
covered pretty much every viable square inch of corporeal real estate. Even I was taken aback by her answer. What had happened to
struggling to say what's wrong with yourself? I was apparently sitting across the desk from the world's most unreluctant self-critic.

Satisfied that she was done, I said, "It's going to take two operations to do it."

She nodded, unfazed, maybe relieved it wasn't going to take, say, *twelve* operations. "I'm widowed a year, and I'm ready to get back out again. I love playing tennis. But I play with a younger group and I don't want to look like the senior one anymore. Can you get me there?"

"I can't guarantee it," I said, "but we'll do everything we can."

On the other hand, one woman of a certain age can personify, all by herself, both the unique strength and beauty of that phase of life, and its cruelty, too. I'm reminded of one of the more haunting photographs I ever saw.

When I was a boy, a woman married an heir to one of the Chicago steel fortunes. Marie was the talk of Lake Forest, as well as of every other suburb in the greater Chicago area. Everyone gossiped even though no one knew much about her—or maybe she was the talk of the town *because* no one knew much about her. She wasn't from Illinois or even the United States. To us, she was, simply, "that Frenchwoman"—beautiful, blond, stylish, charming, vivacious; when she walked into a room, we heard, people noticed. She would become a famous international beauty, married to an American scion.

Years later in New York, after I had established my surgical practice and developed regular contact with the well-connected, I again encountered "that Frenchwoman." In her seventies now, she was still beautiful, stylish, and charming. (She also had extensive sun damage to the face and hands.) She and I talked about Chicago and Illinois and mutual acquaintances.

Once, while in Paris for consults, I was invited by Marie to her apartment (one of at least eight residences she owned). As I walked toward the living room, I passed an impressive Empire-style bureau in the foyer. On it was a framed photograph from the late 1960s that I'll never forget. Marie, maybe forty-five in the picture, is on the arm of her husband, the steel magnate, her partner of some twenty years. They are about to enter Buckingham Palace for a state dinner. She looks magnificent: smiling, slender, radiant. She wears an amethyst-colored evening gown. She looks as beautiful as any woman I've ever seen, an equal to Grace Kelly.

"What an incredible photograph," I said. I knew it was taken at the pinnacle of her husband's power and of her beauty.

"Not so bad," she replied.

"Don't you think you look fabulous?"

"Possibly." She paused. "You know, Robert left me three weeks after the picture was taken for that, that, that . . . how do you say . . . ?" She was too proper to finish the sentence. "And he married her!"

Marie is not alone in her bitterness. (A year later, she was in New York and invited me for cocktails at her Fifth Avenue penthouse. When I asked if it was all right for me to bring the woman I was then dating, she said, "If you're coming with someone, then don't come at all!" and slammed the phone down.)

But because of improved diets, exercise regimens, and economic independence, divorcées and widows I work on are more often than not high-energy and fun. At least half of the older divorcées I know initiated the split, and the vast majority claim that their new, unattached life is more satisfying than their previous existence. They derive particular satisfaction from their work, children and grandchildren, friends, and social lives.

Indeed, while I can't say if the sample of older women patients I see is any kind of a representative cross section, I do know that they are a particularly active and self-starting bunch. After all, they find themselves across the desk from me because they've finally grown so tired of some problem that any obstacle that plastic surgery once represented—it's artificial, it's giving in, it's scary, it's expensive, it's embarrassing—is suddenly an obstacle no longer. They clearly want to take control of some problem, all these recently divorced and separated and widowed women. Yes, for some it's a realization that they once again need to trade on their looks, and if they're going to compete with other women for men, then they want to do so looking as good as they can. For others, it's not about men, but just their own sense of possibility and vitality.

Perhaps the woman who best embodies all these notions rolled into one is Elizabeth, a successful beauty executive in her midseventies, who stopped by my office six days after her face-lift. I thought it was just a happy visit until she showed me the more-than-normal bruising in front of her ear and along the corner of her mouth.

"Hmm," I said, trying to diagnose a cause—but before I proffered an explanation, she solved the mystery.

"We had kinky sex," she said. "My partner couldn't wait any longer so he flipped me over a chair. So I was in the . . . down position for a while there. Which I guess I shouldn't have done."

She smiled.

There is some information I don't need to know.

My Method

▼ ▼ ▼

I have tried to set myself apart in my approach to plastic surgery. I know this approach differs from that of some of my colleagues because patients who've been to other top surgeons have said as much. With many plastic surgeons, the consult walks in, the surgeon looks her over, and he makes his evaluation based on what she looks like in one particular light setting. Not me. When a consult sits down, it's just the first of multiple ways I look at her. First, I evaluate her in my exam room in which fluorescent lights have been positioned strategically so that, as I circle the patient, evaluating her face and neck, I get to see all the shadows and contours. Because it's not just the muscles in our face that are dynamic and that need to be looked at from various angles; our physical world is dynamic, too, not static, and that also affects how the face is perceived. How deep is the shadow cast by the nasolabial fold? How much drooping of the nose is there? Does it cause more shadow in certain light? These are questions anyone might want answered about her face (it might affect what you wear, or how you apply makeup), but it's particularly relevant to someone having surgery, who is making herself over, who is preparing to be out and about again. Are the eyebrows really too low or is the bone protruding too much? I'm looking for nuances. I've trained my eyes to perceive normally, in color, and then almost to switch to perceiving in black and white, to get a starker feel. I'll look at the fine lines in the face in context of the bigger lines. Does the lower lip cast a shadow on the sublabial fold (the area just below the lip that's almost always in slight to substantial shadow)? Does the jaw cast a shadow? Does the cheek cast a shadow? Is there a hollow in the cheek? Then I look closely at the skin—its texture and contour, because that will also affect my evaluation, and thus how I do the surgery. I'll go from "looking" at her in 3-D to 2-D and back to 3-D: By gauging the face in different depths, I can better "see" the skin's texture. I look carefully at the shadows and contours that have created those depressions and elevations.

I look at how shadows are cast on the neck. After age forty-five, women or men come in to talk about their face, but before the conversation is over, they'll almost invariably say that what *really* bothers them most is their neck. The neck usually goes first. Typically, the pattern is this: Before you turn twenty-five (roughly), the two big vertical platysma muscles in your neck don't sag—*can't* sag—because they're "interdigitated," meaning the little fibers inside the muscles crisscross with each other, forming a strong, single cable, which makes for a smooth neck. After age twenty-five, those fibers start to separate, and a right and a left band form, which eventually leads to sagging.

So when, say, a forty-seven-year-old consult sits down, I know generally what's been going on with her anatomy, because that's what's been going on with the anatomy of pretty much everyone her age. But I also know that I'm seeing her at just this one point in time—in the "present tense," if you will. I need to see her in the past tense, too, so I can do a better job at creating her future tense. That's why I ask to see old pictures of her, starting as far back as her twenties. I study the photos with her first, then by myself later. And our actual discussion of the pictures is important, too, because there are nuances to her anatomy that I might pick up on only when hearing her describe them. Were her lips fuller once? How were her breasts then—that is, they sagged less, of course, but how much fuller were they? Maybe that doesn't come out in the photos she's given me, but she'll surely mention it, with some sense of yearning.

(As other surgeons do, I'll also ask the patient to bring in photos she likes, of the feature in question; so a rhinoplasty patient should bring in images of noses she admires, and I'll also have an extensive set of pre- and postnosejob photos that we go through together.)

I don't do computer imaging, for two reasons. First, I don't think it works. It suggests to the patient that the possibilities are close to unlimited, and they aren't; the image you're getting on-screen is still a two-dimensional rendering masquerading as a three-dimensional representation. More often than not, then, it implies a result that's not realistic. I get better results working from photographs, taken at different angles and over time. Second, computer imaging is time-consuming and expensive—so much that I would basically have to hire someone to do it for me.

I look at the patient's face for asymmetry. I know I'll never achieve a perfect symmetry, nor would I want to: Symmetrical faces are boring. Our brains and eye movements are trained not to spend lots of time on forms that are symmetrical; if you mean to catch someone's interest, dress or decorate yourself in a slightly asymmetrical way. In fact, our affinity for asymmetry guides my decision in hiding scars. When I design incisions near the ears for face-lifts, I measure and make certain that they are as symmetrical as possible. The same is true for incisions under the chin when performing chin implants, and for bilateral incisions.

While the face and neck are the areas I most love to work on, I have also done thousands of breast augmentations. (For most surgeons, breast reductions are a smaller percentage of breast procedures performed.) Once again, my philosophy differs from that of many of my colleagues.

The normal shape of the top half of a woman's breast is concave, the bottom half convex. I am not taking credit for this observation. But this shape, as it exists in nature, has quite literally been turned upside down—or at least the upper half has. Now, it's all the rage to put a breast implant underneath the pectoralis muscle, which creates a convex look all the way around; it appears "puffed" because the muscles need time to relax. To me, it looks like a swollen balloon.

Great breast augmentation is best when it fits a woman's body—that is, her chest is proportional to her hips and pelvis. That way, the implant doesn't look obvious, but you can still have great breasts. It is beyond strange to me that several high-profile young actresses I see pictured in magazines want their implants to be visible. They go to movie premieres not just with their breasts pushed up—we expect that—but with the border of the implant visible, either in the center of the chest, when their breasts are pushed together, or on the side, when they wear a dress cut to reveal that.

When doing implants, I have to be almost as careful about cutting as I do with the face, because it's a bad place to have a scar. Women express different preferences for where they want the scars—some want them in the armpit, some around the areola, some underneath where the breasts meet the chest. Preferences vary according to individual, background, and size of breast desired. Putting the scars around the areolas has two significant drawbacks: The accuracy of a mammogram might be compromised, and calcium can get into the scar. One disadvantage of armpit scars is that they may be visible enough to keep the patient from wearing a halter top or strapless dress. New data also indicate that armpit scars may interfere with lymph drainage, which could be especially problematic if the patient develops breast cancer; her treatment may be compromised. Scars, then, must be positioned with care.

Even my patient population for breast augmentation seems to be different from that of my colleagues. I probably see more college-educated women, who tend on average to want smaller implants. My average patient (insofar that anyone can be called an "average" patient) might want to go from a small B to a B, so the size still fits her torso. Big implants, these women often believe, make them look heavy, fat, cheap. However, some women, after coming in for a consultation, won't schedule me because they don't share my aesthetic.

This is where taste—and perhaps subtlety—comes into play.

If a woman has had a breast augmentation and returns to her surgeon, it's almost always because she wants to get still bigger. Only once have I had a returning breast augmentation patient say that I had made her too big.

If I were to err, I would want it to be on the big side. Why? When breast augmentation is performed, a pocket for the implant is formed. This pocket is called a capsule, and it consists of collagen, which contracts around the implant. If an implant is removed altogether, the collagen will retract and the body will reabsorb it completely; if an implant is replaced by a smaller one, the capsule will contract around the new implant and no further dissection is required. However, if an implant is replaced with a bigger one, the pocket must be made larger, which requires more dissection.

After twenty years in solo surgical practice, I have also come up with other techniques that yield results that make my patients. New ways to "feather" fat when doing liposuction so it looks smoother. Cauterizing blood vessels to reduce the dried blood in the wound so that there's less bruising and scarring. A better understanding of perforators—the little arteries that lead off of major blood vessels but which aren't fully described in anatomy books, and whose variability you learn about from hundreds of operations (e.g., I have learned it's better to dissect around perforators rather than to cut them—as others often do—because it allows me to maintain blood flow so that the wound heals faster). I have an understanding of the subtleties of skin, and how it heals differently in a forty-year-old versus a sixty-year-old, in a woman versus a man, and in different places on the body (e.g., the upper eyelid has the best-healing skin on the body).

I am a better surgeon now than I was five years ago, and I expect to be a better one five years from now.

Yet, while saying that a surgeon is skilled and experienced is nice, it's not the ultimate compliment.

He's good with his hands?

A virtue, to be sure, but not the crowning one.

Everyone knows his work?

Massages the ego, but hardly the ultimate compliment.

I trust him?

That's it. The best thing a patient can say about her doctor. I trust him.

You have to be able to tell him exactly what's bothering you and feel that he understands. When he tells you what he thinks you should do, and why, and how he proposes to do it, you should be comfortable with every aspect of it. You must feel he's doing what's best for you, and not because—as happens sometimes with the top-heavy-breast implant surgeons and the ski-jump-nosejob surgeons and the pull-the-skin-until-you-can't-pull-it-anymore face-lift surgeons—it's what *he* thinks looks good, or because it's the only look he knows how to do well.

Trust is vital for a simpler reason: *You're having surgery*. If something should happen while you're under, and your surgeon needs to make a quick, unanticipated decision, you want that decision made by a person not only of unsurpassed competency, but whose priorities and aesthetic match yours.

I was Alma's second surgeon. Her first, an extremely reputable surgeon in Washington, D.C., had done a breast augmentation. The implants were a little too big for her. At five feet five, with a medium frame and narrow hips, her chest was slightly out of proportion. While I agreed with her that the implants didn't fit her frame, it was hardly egregious, and I told her so. When she said they made her look fat, I disagreed. (I would have told her otherwise had I thought so. While I don't relish telling a patient she looks heavy, it's my job to be as objective as she needs me to be.)

What bothered her more than what everyone could see, however, was what only she (or an intimate) could see, something that had bothered her since she was a preteen: her large areolas. There was nothing irregular about them; they were part of her normal anatomy. But when the other surgeon had put in her implants, he hadn't proposed reducing the size of the areolas, nor had she been forceful enough to bring it up. Once the implants were in, the areolas looked even bigger, verging on misshapen.

The net result of the implants? She was more unhappy than before the surgery.

I could see what a relief it was for her to get her whole story out. She acknowledged that she liked her breasts to look big, and she almost liked the size of the new implants. But her larger, asymmetrical areolas made her feel ugly and unfeminine.

After I looked at her breasts, we decided to reduce the areolas considerably, to a diameter of three inches, down from six inches, and also to reduce the size of the implants by one size. To do the former, I would draw a circle around each areola, draw an inner circle of the desired size, then remove the encircled skin, widely undermine the normal breast skin, and close the circle by bringing the outer skin surface to the inner, or areolar, surface.

Alma was anesthetized and I began. I reduced the areolas down to a size that looked great. At three inches, they were pretty, normal, and feminine, and I was optimistic that they would make her happy . . . but now I realized she looked best with no implants at all. In fact, in listening carefully to her intimate monologue about how she'd felt about her breasts from puberty, I deduced that much of the image she had of herself, and much of what drove the image she wanted to present to the world, had to do with her unhappiness about what was underneath, specifically her areolas. And if she was happy with what was underneath, then it followed that she would see that her normal breast size was absolutely fine and attractive for her body type.

So reducing the implants by one size—which we'd agreed on—was not enough. I felt that if I followed that route, she wouldn't be happy afterward—*happier,* yes, but not happy. Big difference. Yet I couldn't wake her to get her approval. During the consult, I hadn't said to her, *So, Alma, if I reduce the areolas and then I realize that we need to reduce the breast volume even more than we'd thought, I'm going to do that, okay?* I just went ahead and did what I knew was right, knowing all that she'd confided in me, and that she trusted my judgment, aesthetically and medically.

I removed the implants. Altogether.

Alma was asleep when I made this independent decision, but it wasn't *really* made independently. While as a surgeon I make judgments about what's best for my patient, when there's trust and rapport, the decisions aren't hard to make.

Alma awoke. When she was alert, I gave her a mirror to get a good look at her new implant-free, smaller-areola breasts.

In my entire career as a surgeon, I have never had a happier patient.

Or a happier significant other. Days later, Alma's husband came by the office with Alma to express his gratitude. While husbands always—or so I'd thought—want their wives to have bigger breasts, this case was different.

"Thank you so much," he said, shaking both of my hands and tearing up. "It's not that she's more beautiful to me, because that's not possible. But now my wife knows just how beautiful is the woman I've been looking at for fourteen years."

Men

▼ ▼ ▼

George, a divorced, balding investment banker who'd worked for PaineWebber his entire adult life, retired at sixty-two, then came to see me.

"I've wanted to do my face and nose for twenty years," he said. "I woke up every day thinking about it. But I was afraid to walk into work on Monday after having a face-lift."

It was sad and it wasn't. He confessed to thinking he was over the hill, and that life for him was finished—yet here he was in my office, obviously trying to do something about it. Plus, he said, he'd met a younger woman.

"Between her and you," he said. "Maybe that'll be my ticket to youth."

I was pleased for the opportunity but I had my work cut out. Not only was George totally bald but he had low eyebrows. How was I going to pull this off without large, visible scars across the top of his head? He didn't want to wear a toupee. I had to tell him that nothing would really return his youth. But I could make him look better, despite the apparent difficulty.

I told George about a new procedure, an endoscopic browlift, suited for hiding scars, but I still couldn't guarantee him a great result. The scars would be in the front part of the skull, at the top of the scalp, I told him; how visible they would be, I couldn't say. At that point in my practice, I'd done few endoscopic browlifts, all on men with hair.

George told me to go for it.

Three weeks later, before he'd even entered the office to have the sutures removed, I was cringing. How would George look once the stitches were removed?

I didn't have to worry. Not only would the scars turn out to be practically invisible, but George entered my office with his new wife, the younger woman he'd been seeing. He'd married her during the first week post-op—a fairly persuasive argument that, even before the bruising is gone, the happier psychology brought about by a cosmetic surgical procedure has taken root.

While in 2003, according to the American Society of Plastic Surgeons, men underwent only 14 percent of total cosmetic procedures, their total numbers had jumped nearly 30 percent from just the previous year. Lip augmentation for men increased by 740 percent; upper-arm lifts, 606 percent; buttock lifts, 554 percent; thigh lifts, 147 percent; and chin augmentation, 70 percent . . . *in just one year*. Among nonsurgical, minimally invasive procedures, Botox injections for men, over the previous year, increased 152 percent; microdermabrasion, 87 percent; cellulite treatment, 71 percent; and laser treatment of leg veins, 42 percent. Part of this increase is due to the diminished stigma of plastic surgery, part is due to innovations that allow for quicker recovery time and less fussing, and part is due to the continually growing pressure to look young longer for the sake of professional advancement. But increasing numbers of men, like George, come to me simply because they want to look better, not because they're terrified of getting passed over for promotion. (The difference between the percentage of men who get cosmetic surgery for largely professional reasons and the percentage of women who do so is narrowing, at least among my patient sample.)

Today, 15 percent of my patients are men. The most popular procedure I do on them is a necklift. Mid-face-lifts represent a considerably smaller part of my surgeries. Lots of men want rhinoplasties and eye lifts. Liposuction for hips and stomach are also popular. I've never done a male tummy tuck.

Lots of surgeons don't like doing face-lifts on men. Male skin is less pliable. Men have a greater concentration of blood vessels in the face than women do, making us more prone to bruising. Postoperatively, I advise men to wrap their faces a little tighter than I advise for women, and men need to be more disciplined about applying ice for the first forty-eight hours. Our hair follicles go deeper, all the way into the subcutaneous level of fat, and our hair distribution must be considered: Most men don't have hair in front of or right behind their ears. When doing a full face-lift (as opposed to a browlift) on a man, particularly a balding or bald man, I make my incisions inside the ear or right behind it. I might also leave some extra skin to cover an incision, or, where possible, shorten the scar. With a woman, I can go for a smoother face and neck, because scars are easier to hide.

Men decide faster than women what they want. Of course there are variations within each sex. But when Typical Guy comes into the office, he knows exactly what he wants.

Can you do it? he asks. *What are the risks? How much does it cost?*

I tell him the good and the bad. He makes up his mind right there in the office.

When can you do it? he asks.

I tell him. He leaves.

In the days before the operation, he rarely calls. He almost never complains. Afterward, when it's done, it's done.

Women second-guess themselves much more, both in the consultation and in the days before surgery. "Should I make it a 34C?" says a woman who seemed sure she wanted a 36B. Or: "Should I do my nose, too?" Almost no woman makes up her mind yes or no while sitting in the consultation, unless I'm the third or fourth surgeon she's visited and she's decided to go with me.

Women also want to tell a story. "There's this role I want to play," began one actress, and described the character, the character's backstory, the play, her favorite role in high school, and her sister's recent conversion to born-again Christianity before getting to what it was about her face and body that she'd come about. (Ten minutes later, she got to the punch line: "Can you reduce this scar?") Other women will talk about a skirt or blouse that they love but have stopped wearing because of this or that flaw. They'll provide lots of personal history. I listen.

George notwithstanding, men almost never talk about their life.

Some of my most fulfilling moments occur when husbands call to thank me. It's usually about a month after the procedure. The men are pleased with their wife's new appearance.

But not all.

In this case, the husband was calling to complain.

"Thanks a lot, Doctor," he said edgily. "You broke up my marriage."

"Excuse me?" I said.

He told me that a month before, I had done breast augmentation on his wife—a gift from him to her. One day months earlier, he had commented on the smallish size of her chest, and she had not let him forget it.

After the surgery, her attitude about everything in the marriage changed. Instead of her appreciating his gift, he said, she appreciated nothing about him. And said so.

She left him.

"It's your fault," he told me on the phone.

That's the exception, though. Mostly, men will express gratitude to me for anything from a revised scar to a small lipo to an eyelid lift on their partner. The men tell me that their wife is happier and more confident, and the husbands are reaping the benefits of the improved state of mind.

Husbands rarely accompany their spouse to plastic surgery. So when they do, it's a nice change. One morning, a handsome couple in their forties came in. She wanted a face-lift. I looked at her, examined her under various lights, told her I would need to see photographs of her when she was younger, then described to her in detail what was involved.

The whole time, her husband sat there, not saying a word, sizing me up.

That afternoon, my office manager, Tanya, told me that the husband was on the phone and wanted to know if he could come in the following day.

Fine, I told Tanya.

The next day, he was back in my office—only this time accompanying his Dutch girlfriend, who wanted a breastlift.

After the consult, the man took me aside and said he knew he didn't have to tell me (or my staff) to schedule the surgeries on different days.

Gay men, on the whole, want the same procedures as straight men except for two differences: They sometimes ask for lipo when they don't really need it, and they're more likely to come in for multiple procedures. They want eye lifts, nosejobs, and liposuction, usually for the stomach. My gay clientele is particularly high-profile and accomplished, made up of movie directors, artists, actors, advertising men, and doctors.

If there's one patient demographic—a rather narrowly defined one—that I can now say is almost guaranteed to be unhappy with their operation, it's narcissistic gay men who come in for nasal surgery. They're unhappy with themselves beforehand; they invariably express deep unhappiness with the procedure afterward.

On the other hand, it's hard to find a patient easier to satisfy than Richard, a top advertising executive who, upon being introduced to me at a cocktail party, listed, at full volume, all the procedures he could use.

"God, I really need to have my eyes done!" he said. "And lipo my hips, please! And maybe a little neck work? Could we do that?"

Anyone speaking so boldly about cosmetic surgery, I thought, was probably not completely serious about it, so I didn't expect to see Richard again. But three months later he showed up at my office and confirmed that he wanted all the procedures he'd rattled off.

I described the details of each procedure, then told him the effect would be subtle and that no one would notice.

"No one will notice?" he said. "I don't care if they know! I *want* them to know!"

When it comes to sensitive subjects, a woman will often demur. A man who speaks openly about sensitive things will usually do so in a different tone.

Once, while on a trip to Florida to meet with consults, I took an afternoon to visit an Andover buddy, Kent Vogel, who'd become a fighter pilot and had invited me to Tyndall Air Force Base in the panhandle to watch jet-fighter training. He said the pilots would love it.

"They'll laugh their ass off at a plastic surgeon," said Kent.

I understood what he meant—not that what I did was "sissy" stuff, but that, in some ways, it represented the very opposite of the realm he maneuvered in.

I got security clearance (I found out later that they'd scouted me all the way back to my prep-school days) and was introduced to the colonel, a Vietnam vet in charge of the fighter squadron. He briefly introduced me to the fliers—"The Makos," they called themselves, based out of Homestead, Florida. They'd all been flying since they were maybe sixteen, and they looked like clichés of American fighter pilots. In all my days as a plastic surgeon and circulating among beautiful people, I've never seen a better-looking, sharper bunch of young men.

It happened to be Aerial Dogfight Day, with the exercises designed to prepare the pilots for dogfights. They also constantly entertained the possibility of an enemy jet emerging from Cuban airspace. Before the pilots went up, I watched and listened as they went through their checklists: one for avionics, one for hydraulics, one for power systems, one for armaments. What they did and what I did wasn't so opposite, after all; their preflight preparation reminded me a great deal of what I did preoperatively.

Then the guys went up.

The colonel let me watch the exercises with him from the control room. Looking at the incredibly high-tech instruments all around me, I could see everything going on with each of the jets involved in the exercises—their location, their airspeed, the angle of their bank. I was amazed by the sophistication of the technology. This is what I loved so much about science: Every instrument was an improvement on an instrument that had come before and would help lead to better instruments tomorrow. It was true for plastic surgery and true for fighter jet technology.

On a big screen, I could see the jets—each represented by a knot of constantly changing numbers—maneuvering around each other, and I tried to follow the flight path of my friend Kent, who was up there in the thick of the dogfight. Everything going on in the cockpits was broadcast over the loudspeaker, and the rush of it and the language were exactly as one might imagine.

"He's on my tail!" bellowed one of the pilots over the loudspeaker. *"He's on my tail!"*

The numbers representing the lagging jet swooped in just as the lead jumble of numbers twisted away in a nifty maneuver. They were beautiful machines up there, screaming across the sky.

"He's on your tail, Vogel! Look out!"

The colonel looked at me. "Your friend just got flamed."

Afterward, in the pilots' room, Kent and other members of the squadron sat around talking about what they could have done better. The colonel entered and rubbed his hands together.

"Okay, gentlemen," he barked, "the real reason Dr. Vogel brought in Dr. Lesesne here is because . . . *you're all ugly!*" The colonel went down the line, pilot by pilot, pointing out the allegedly hideous defects of each man's face—this one's nose, that one's hairline, this guy's teeth. The comments were pointed, and somewhat truthful, but generally hilarious, since each guy looked like a young Harrison Ford or at least a cousin of Tom Cruise's.

It was a thrilling day; such a contrast to the tone of my work. It was especially illuminating, even amusing, in reminding me of the vast differences in style and psychology between men and women. Here were two professions, both highly technical, both highly confidential. Here, guys could be heard yelling over loudspeakers; guys were getting "flamed" in front of their colleagues; guys were openly mocking each other's looks (and guys far less good-looking than these men will do the same, I've noticed).

Would any woman ever do that to her girlfriend? *In front of other women?* Might she enjoy being shot down in front of them, or shooting her friends down? And having it broadcast?

Are you nuts?

I'm Ready for My Close-up Now

▼　▼　▼

It's not just that Hollywood embraces cosmetic surgery like no other place on earth—that it's more ubiquitous, more celebrated, more procedures per patient, and it's initiated at a younger age. What's more noteworthy, I think, is that the on-screen talent aren't the only ones who've had plastic surgery. All the entertainment-industry players have had it, too, if they want to be players—directors, writers, and particularly agents and studio executives. An executive at a major movie studio periodically calls to get my opinion on what work I might advise for an actor they're considering to star in a big-budget picture. I'll recommend a procedure or two (or none at all), knowing, as I do now, that the real reason he's calling is to see when I'll be out there again, to work on him and his executive-level buddies.

Corporate Hollywood wants the same procedures as the stars—nose, eyes, lipo, breast implants, cheek implants, and a much higher percentage of injectables than the general population. It makes sense. Their task is to drive film approval, and most of their product is youth-driven films. Many of them feel as if they can't compete professionally in a town based largely on looks if they don't themselves look good.

Yet despite the celebration of plastic surgery in the Hollywood culture, there's still a desire to keep one's surgery secret, on one hand, while on the other, to expose who's had what.

I'd been invited to an awards banquet. I was keeping a doctor's low profile (not hard to do given the star power in the theater) when a director, whom I know socially, sat beside me and gestured at one of America's most popular leading men across the room.

"I would cast him if he weren't such a lush and didn't look like he'd been partying all night long," he said. "Can you make him look less dissipated?"

"Sure," I said.

"How would you do it?"

"The first thing is to make sure he's stopped drinking. Then I'd take the bags out from below his eyes and remove some skin from the upper lids. He could use some neck work, not too much, and liposuction for that belly."

The director—who, while prominent, didn't come close to the clout of the star—seemed to think he might be able to convince the star to come see me.

It didn't happen so fast.

Months later, I noticed heavy retouching of photographs of the star in ads for his new movie. Weeks after that, Tanya said, "There's a call for you from Los Angeles."

It was the star.

He asked if I did Botox. I said yes. But it became apparent to me, from his questions, that he was starting down the road of cosmetic fixes much more major than Botox.

Despite the comment of a woman friend, one of Hollywood's top agents, that "all actresses have work done if they're going to stay in the business; this growing-old-gracefully business is nonsense," it obviously applies to certain types of talent and not others. Pamela Anderson along with many B-list actresses would have different careers had they not had breast augmentation (often more than once). For many of them the decision to have such surgery is extremely justified. For some less ostentatious actresses, plastic surgery can prolong careers or keep the range of their offered parts from narrowing.

Then again, to be believable, a face that has signs of aging should not be totally smooth. If you obliterate all crow's-feet or the nasolabial folds from an aging face, a mask will result, diminishing the ability to express oneself facially. If Meryl Streep or someone of her ilk had such a procedure, it would probably hurt her credibility and thus her career. Actors need to be especially wary of using Botox or fillers to smooth their skin because it results in a flat, affectless face. (I worked on one actress who wanted me to give her Botox "so I look sad," she said. She came back a year later, on the eve of taking another role, asking for Botox in another part of her face "so I look happy.") An actor should improve the contour of the face as it ages and make the pigmentation more homogeneous, and not worry so much about skin texture.

Actors have the right to be pickier than anyone else about plastic surgery. For them, a bad face-lift isn't just demoralizing. It loses them movie roles. It costs them their livelihood. True, fashion models also live off their looks—more singularly than actors, in fact— but models (except for Lauren Hutton and a few others) are invariably long out of the game by forty-two, the age when most people, gorgeous or not, start "needing" work (give or take a few years, depending on genes, sun damage, and cigarette/alcohol/drug consumption).

I take precautions with actors. When I ask for photos, I tell them I don't want head shots, which are almost always retouched. Scheduling is crucial with actors, given long film shoots and particularly the seasonality of TV work. For the biggest stars (and extremely secretive lesser ones), I give them my cell number, something that most high-profile patients prefer (and which all politicians insist on). Leading up to the surgery, the actor or actress often wants to speak only with me, or she might even use a friend as her front person.

When an actor shows up for the surgery, only my anesthesiologist and I know who it is. They'll typically come to the office for a face-lift early Saturday or Sunday morning, usually wearing sunglasses. (This is at my Park Avenue office. While I do initial consults and injectables in L.A., I do most of my Hollywood-related surgery in New York.) Depending on where I perform the operation, afterward the star is driven in a hired car to a "safe hotel" in Santa Monica or Manhattan (a discreet, high-end hotel that has a separate wing). A private-duty nurse will stay with the star for a night. A number of California-based actors actually prefer to have surgery in New York because they believe the medical institutions are, on the whole, better. (I agree: There are more major teaching hospitals in New York, the plastic surgery departments are older, and there's a greater concentration of expertise.)

I find that most major actresses are not the egomaniacs they're often made out to be and can be quite delightful. Because of their livelihood, the first, last, and only determining standard is results. There are excellent plastic surgeons all over Los Angeles and Beverly Hills, and some movie stars have had masterful face-lifts and eye jobs where they're able to keep the same expression year after year. This is especially important when they're making sequels. Sylvester Stallone and Arnold Schwarzenegger may have had too much work. Who knows? What would they have looked like had they had nothing done? The plastic surgery ethos on the West Coast tends to favor shinier, more "obvious" results. Some actors prefer that. Most don't. The popular magazines and tabloids that speculate on stars' possible plastic surgery procedures ignore the pressure on actors to look young for their careers. So while one can criticize an obvious result, people fail to take into account that most actors must do something to stop time, if they want to remain employed.

When I operate on actors, I consider thoroughly that their look will be influenced very much by all kinds of light falling on them. While filming *Around the World in 80 Days,* Shirley MacLaine, then twenty-two, said she learned the most about acting from Marlene Dietrich, age fifty-four, because Dietrich knew how to act "in light"—that is, how to get the cameraman to give her favorable light. (Who can forget Gloria Swanson, as the faded movie star Norma Desmond in *Sunset Boulevard,* delivering her famous line—"All right, Mr. DeMille, I'm ready for my close-up"—as she approaches the camera with her head tilted ever so slightly to one side, her good one?) When I was an on-air health consultant for NBC News, the one piece of advice I remember was *Make friends with the cameraman to get good lighting.* American history might be very different if Richard Nixon had learned that simple lesson.

When I'm evaluating actors in my office, I'm hyperaware of lighting. I swing them around into different shadings and intensities of light, turn their head, look at them as light is coming in from oblique angles, from above, from below. For a face-lift, I may decide to leave a little fold or a little more fat than I would take out with a nonactor, knowing that that extra skin may be needed to cover an incision, which could make a difference in a close-up.

A couple of years ago, a stage actress well known for her character roles on Broadway came to see me. She was in her seventies—a young seventy, though—and made sure that I understood that, whatever youth-restoring improvements I made to her face, I was not to overdo it. She wanted still to be considered for the wide range of parts she was frequently offered—late fifties to seventy. In other words, she wanted to look younger but not *that* much younger.

Definitely not "pulled." While other women her age have told me to make them look as young as possible, for Michelle her driving motivation was to maintain her professional viability. When I did the face-lift, I left a little skin around her jawline, did not pull her neck as tight as I might otherwise have, and did not add quite as much fat to her lips.

I fly to L.A. every two months, for two to three days—a couple days of consults, Botox and injectables, possibly surgery, and a day of seeing friends. I have a relationship with a hotel there and use one of their suites for my meetings. For my patients' protection, I may register under a pseudonym to fend off gossip-magazine snoops. Sometimes I'll meet my high-profile consults on Ocean Drive in Santa Monica. I'll wait by a little park above Pacific Coast Highway, they'll come walking along, and then we'll walk side by side—very postwar Berlin. Walking north, they'll tell me what they want; when we turn around and head south toward the pier, I'll tell them what I can do. I especially like meeting this way because I get to see them in natural sunlight.

Holly, forty-five, a major actress, was my first appointment on one of my visits.

I rarely watch TV, go to the movies or the theater. So it was not until later that I discovered just how well known and successful Holly was, a rare triple threat: TV, film, and Broadway, big-time projects in all three media. She had several Emmy and Tony nominations to her credit (she won one) and created a defining role in one of America's most popular film comedies. But I might have guessed she was a star anyway (either that or she would have to be delusional) because when she entered my hotel suite, she had on a blond wig, sunglasses, and a long coat. And in what I would come to see as a stroke of disguise ingenuity, she wore flats. Why was that ingenious? So any nosy people who might spot her would not suspect it was her, because she was short. Holly (I later found out) always wears high heels in public. *Always.* Wouldn't be caught dead in flats—precisely to fight off the impression that she's very short. Meeting me in flats, then, she would appear her natural *short* short self—ergo, unrecognizable.

Give people credit for thinking these things out.

On our first encounter, I liked her immediately. She was very attractive—great figure, good legs, had worked out her whole life. She had lines on her face but they were not inappropriate. She didn't have lots of hanging skin and jowl. And she exuded great sex appeal—which, to me, is all about animation and movement. She walked in a way that was alluring, not provocative. When she took a seat, it was in a feminine, stylish way. She was quick to smile. With some of the women I operate on, the older they get, the *greater* their sex appeal, and it lasts well into their sixties and even beyond. Holly, with a twinkle in her eye, was one of those whose sex appeal would continue for years.

I could see she'd had surgery done on her face. But Holly wanted something done to her eyebrows, and she absolutely did *not* want her hairline pulled back. I promised her we could accomplish what she wanted by eschewing a whole face-lift and doing a short-scar browlift, which focuses on the eyebrows and wouldn't cost her a single hair follicle. I would make tiny incisions in the scalp, dissecting and releasing the skin that allows the eyebrows to go up, then elevating that skin and affixing it in a higher position. She nodded. I asked her when she would like the surgery.

She was "between movies," she said, "so my window of time is now." She did not say it in a prima donna way. (And given the number of movies she'd made, the phrase *between movies* seemed a matter-of-fact description, not actorspeak for "it's doubtful I'll ever be in another movie.")

I told her I thought I could get OR time in a couple of days.

Immediately after the surgery, I thought she looked unbelievable. Unfortunately, she didn't share that opinion. She was anxious about her new look, a typical reaction so soon after the operation. But a short-scar browlift heals relatively quickly, and the bruising is usually limited, along the hairline.

Her husband rushed over to see Holly and called me to say that he was floored, in a good way. Still, Holly was not persuaded.

She invited me to accompany her to dinner three nights later, perhaps to convince herself she looked better (or maybe to taunt me, if she still hated the results). I was planning to still be in L.A. then so I said yes. At the restaurant, we dined with several people, and to them and the many others who stopped by the table, she introduced me (I was impressed to witness) as a plastic surgeon—though not *her* plastic surgeon.

I was amazed. What had happened to the woman in the film noir disguise?

Then I figured it out. This was a clever woman, a worldly and smart woman. She had convinced the world she was not that short, after all, so she could hide in it by being very short. And now this was another clever move, a test of her own devising.

What she was doing, I surmised, was to see how many of the people who were introduced to me would put two and two together. As an actress, she was good at reading authentic reactions.

After all, what person in show business would actually introduce her plastic surgeon?

No one appeared to take the bait. Then again, several of those I was introduced to were themselves actors, so maybe they were just as good at *hiding* their reactions.

Holly was happy. Her test was successful. Suddenly, I had done a good job.

It was another example of how you must always accomplish

two things: *Do* make the patient look good; *don't* make it obvious why she looks good.

Holly would come to see me two years later for a second operation, arm liposuction, and this time she showed up for the consult undisguised.

The third time I saw her, a year after that, was in Palm Springs. Holly called to ask if I would meet her by the hotel pool. At a conversational volume—no whispering—she told me she wanted a necklift. I nodded that, yes, I thought it might be time.

"Do you want me to show you what I'm thinking?" I asked quietly.

"Yes," she said.

I stood. "Would you like to go inside, away from so many—"

"No. Here is fine."

I hesitated for a second. She nodded as if to say, *It's all right.*

I nodded back. I held her hair away from her neck, looked at it in front of her ears and behind. I was discreet—that's the essence of our work, after all—but still: We were by a resort swimming pool, where industry people came and went. It was stunning how much more comfortable Holly had become with the idea of plastic surgery. Indeed, if I wasn't mistaken, there might even have been a bit of pride-taking in me, in *her* plastic surgeon, not just any plastic surgeon. She'd come to trust me so much, she seemed to be inviting the exposure.

Perhaps this is what psychoanalysts experience, I thought, when their patients experience "transference." As for me, while it was a bit of an ego stroke to have this movie star clearly enjoy being around me, I'd just as soon stay behind the scenes.

I try to see as many L.A. patients as I can when I'm there. I always enjoy the chance to meet people on their turf, especially in their home. After my initial meeting with Holly, I was invited to the "bungalow" of a very famous movie actor. I drove my rental car along the winding road down into Topanga Canyon. I almost missed the turnoff onto the isolated road where he lived. The house was gated, with two guards outside. When I got inside, though, Billy was standing outside his door to greet me—no butler or maid or entourage. He was down-to-earth and easygoing. He was not considered a dramatic actor but an action-film guy, and he'd enjoyed one of the longer runs in Hollywood. He'd also had too much skin and fat taken out of his lower lids and had small scars visible near his ears.

We sat in his living room facing each other. The dynamic of the virgin encounter between patient and surgeon can be quite amusing—patient scanning doctor's face and eyes for trustworthiness and a glint of competency; doctor scanning patient's face and eyes to see what procedures need to be done, and how good the results could be. But it was heightened here, partly because it was in his home, partly because it was man-to-man, partly because he wasn't a novice. He'd had two procedures done before, he said. This time he knew what he wanted—not to look younger (he was in his early sixties) but to look more natural.

We continued to size each other up. He didn't waste words. He reminded me of the old movie cowboys who speak not a syllable more than necessary. The actor took out old photos of himself. Even though I had noticed his waxier complexion right away (anyone would have, as I'm sure his moviegoing audience had, too), I was shocked at just how unnatural he seemed now. The browlift he'd had made him look startled, and he'd had surgery to reduce the muscles in his forehead—odd for an actor, I thought, since it compromised his expressiveness. It would have been cruel and pointless to tell him how awful the previous surgeries had been.

"Your job," he said, his finger pointing at me like a gun. "Make me look natural again." There was a touch of sadness in his eyes and voice, but it was still well short of desperation.

When I left, I had no idea what he thought of me or what he would decide; maybe that was the actor in him. But I suspected I would not hear back. Straight shooter though he seemed, I felt he'd become fatigued by what plastic surgery had done to him. Enough was enough.

Six months later, he called. "Woulda called sooner," he said. "Shot a movie." I was glad to see he was as true as I'd first thought.

"New York, next week," he said. "Book me. Lots of drugs, Cap."

Not surprisingly, he showed up at my office alone, just sunglasses and hat as cover. And they might not have been cover: It was a sunny, cool New York day.

Some actors say they don't want to be noticed, even though they come with an entourage. Or they'll profess their love of anonymity, then have front-row seats at the theater and make sure to stand and face the audience and pretend they're looking for someone right before the lights go down, so everyone can get a look.

And some actors really, truly don't need to be noticed, nor do they have to announce to the world that they don't need it. Billy was one of those.

Two years later, at the end of a busy day and with the waiting room finally empty, my office manager, Tanya, poked her head in my office.

"There's a Robert Walker here to see you," she said. I asked her to show him in.

It was Billy, looking fifteen years younger, accompanied by a younger woman.

"Cap, my friend?" he said. "This is Susan from Chicago. Susan, Cap. She liked the way you made me look. She wants to talk to you about her eyes."

Sometimes you take risks. Some actresses come with the reputation for being difficult. With Stella, an actress who had costarred on a successful TV crime drama, I knew if I didn't get it exactly right (by her standards), my name would be smeared across Beverly Hills and Los Angeles.

I did a browlift on her and she was . . . dissatisfied! How shocking!

"This is not what I had in mind," she said to me glumly on my cell phone, not two hours after the procedure. "This is . . . this is . . . this is gonna be a *big* problem."

I pointed out to Stella that it had been all of ninety minutes since the operation was over. I tried to get her to articulate what was upsetting her. She just kept repeating ominously, "This is gonna be a *big* problem." When I tried once more to get a specific complaint from her, she said she had another call coming in and cut me off.

Damn, I thought. I should have known better.

Fortunately, this is Hollywood.

The nature of actors is such that the final judgment on certain big career decisions doesn't always lie with them. Stella's husband loved the face-lift. More important, Stella's agent, manager, and publicist all loved it.

Ergo, Stella loved it.

Stella called back a week later to say she was now happy, and when she needed surgery in the future, she'd be calling me.

Which reminds me of a favorite Hollywood story someone told me: Writer gives script to Producer. After the weekend, Writer calls Producer. "Did you read it?"

"Yes," Producer answers.

"And?"

"I don't know."

"What do you mean you don't know?" asks Writer.

"No one *else* has read it," says Producer, "so I don't know what I think yet."

Failures
(and What to Ask a Surgeon)
▼ ▼ ▼

It's one of the more common questions: Why is there so much awful plastic surgery and injectable work among actresses and actors who can afford anything? Even big stars can have trouble finding the right person. A major, Emmy Award–winning actress went to a reputable Los Angeles surgeon for an upper-eyelid lift, and he was reluctant to do what he thought was best because she was stage-directing his every suggestion. It turned out to be a total failure. He took out all the skin she wanted—and it made the eyelid lag open at night, exposing the cornea.

Why did the problem happen? She had done her homework and had found a competent surgeon—that's a positive—but there was no rapport between them, and he merely followed her directions rather than taking charge. The same thing happened to me and a Hollywood producer: She came to me and dictated what she wanted done with her face-lift. It was early in my career. She visited me six times before we did the procedure. But I should have said—and do say now, in similar circumstances—*No. Hold on. That won't look good.* I wanted to do more than she did; she said, *Don't do this . . . don't do that*. She dictated to me.

Sure enough, she was unhappy that I didn't pull her more.

My advice? See a surgeon you trust, spend time with him, and if he has a solution, you should do it his way. And if he doesn't think a particular procedure is advisable, you probably shouldn't insist.

▼

Bad work is going to happen, for a variety of reasons. Fortunately, in many cases, things can be done to remedy the problem.

A wealthy, sixty-three-year-old Chicagoan had undergone a face-lift during which two facial nerves were cut, so that she had lost almost half the facial control of her eyelids and smile. Her eyes drooped and she drooled. She disappeared from sight, jetting to Paris (where she had an apartment) so that her closest friends couldn't see her. When she discussed her plight with an acquaintance, she was referred to me (I had done a face-lift on the Parisian) and paid me a visit. Six procedures later, I had reconstructed her eyelid so that it didn't droop and her mouth so she wouldn't drool. A nerve can sometimes be repaired, but at her age I was not confident it would succeed. Instead, I fixed the symptoms by transferring muscle from the scalp, and using sutures to support the drooping muscles. She was better but not perfect. Unfortunately, the facial nerve paralysis is permanent.

There's a risk in taking on the job of fixing poor results. If you succeed, you get to be the hero. But if you try to correct a disaster and fail (e.g., it's just so bad to begin with), the distraught patient will often blame you *more* than the original doctor. You're the one most immediately associated with the problem, and you may have compounded it. They only remember the last operation.

It's the alpha and omega of the Hippocratic oath, its golden rule:

Primum non nocere. First, do no harm.

Laudable and commonsensical. An admonition all doctors should heed. But sometimes results don't meet expectations—the doctor's or the patient's. Sometimes the problem is unavoidable.

And sometimes it's the doctor's fault. Not long ago, a twenty-year-old woman undergoing a breast augmentation had a respiratory obstruction and went into cardiac arrest. An unlicensed nurse anethetist in the room could not control the airway; the surgeon's operating room was not certified.

Or this Westchester case, just as disturbing: The patient had apparently not come out of anesthesia for nine hours...at which time the surgeon was finally able to bring himself to tell her family that she'd gone into cardiac arrest, and died, five hours before.

These disasters happen very rarely when a competent, well-trained surgeon is involved.

Although it's hard to find a positive to terrible stories like this (particularly, of course, for the families of the patients involved), our medical system is set up to make catastrophes less prevalent. Each hospital is required to use a "morbidity/mortality" reporting system, whereby people are motivated to report problems so that our medical institutions can investigate what went wrong and safety is enhanced. Situations like the ones above are, as a matter of routine, brought up by the hospital's quality assurance program. Such systems are meant to oversee medical disasters and mishaps the way the FAA oversees flight disasters and mishaps.

Yet it distresses me when bad results happen, particularly if the physician involved doesn't care, is untrained, or abandons the patient. And I mean real disasters, not ones where the patient and doctor have a different perception of the color of the scars. I'm distressed first, of course, for the patient who's been hurt. Then I'm distressed because it reflects badly upon doctors and surgeons. In the last couple of years, there have been a number of high-profile plastic surgery disasters. Some of the more publicized disasters include the death of a forty-two-year-old Irish woman, following a rhinoplasty performed by an ENT surgeon who'd had his license restricted; bilateral facial paralysis, requiring ICU hospitalization, after a patient was given home-made Botox; death after lipo by an oral surgeon; cardiac arrest during a face-lift at a dentist's office. The disasters by these physicians or dentists are all too common and not surprising, considering the training involved, or their demeanor.

Sometimes a problem is the result of patient factors. For example, procedures involving a patient who smokes have a higher complication rate. One prominent Dallas plastic surgeon simply won't operate on smokers. I believe that you can, but you have to tailor your operation and expectations accordingly. Smoking can lead to wounds healing badly, poor scars, and increased pigmentation. Breastlifts and face-lifts are particularly problematic for smokers because in both cases there's a need for skin elevation. Skin is elevated to a new place and will survive only if blood reaches it. So good blood flow is vital; nicotine interferes with that.

In some instances, the result could have been surgically prevented had the patient only done her homework and stayed away from that surgeon or practitioner.

But how does a patient, particularly a first-timer, know what to ask and look for? To increase your chance for a good experience with plastic surgery, here are some steps to take and questions to ask—both before you pick a doctor and then once you're sitting in his or her office.

1. Contact the American Society of Plastic Surgeons (888-4PLASTIC; www.plasticsurgery.org), our professional organization. Ask for a brochure on the procedure you're considering. Even though the procedure may not address concerns specific to you (your age, genetics, goal, etc.), and

the ASPS may slightly overplay the severity of the
procedure, it's a good place to start.

2. Ask friends or local doctors for plastic surgeons they
recommend.

3. Once you have names, check to see if they're board-certified.
Virtually every week, I see at least one patient in my office
because of a bad result from a non-board-certified plastic
surgeon, and I see it from every part of the country (and
often these surgeons came recommended).

    Whose board am I talking about? The American Board of
Plastic Surgery (ABPS). That one, and only that one. While
other boards exist, in my opinion they do not require the
same rigorous training or follow-up after training. I should
say here that I'm partial to plastic surgeons. I believe that
when it comes to doing cosmetic surgery, they do the best job
(compared with dermatologists, ear-nose-and-throat doctors,
oral surgeons, dentists, ob-gyns, orthopedic surgeons, and
nurses who may also perform certain cosmetic procedures).
Our training is usually longer, more arduous, and the
scrutiny we receive from our professional organizations,
after we complete our training, is second to none.

    To check on a surgeon's board certification, call the ABPS
in Philadelphia (215-587-9322; www.abplsurg.org) or the
ASPS. They can tell you not only if surgeons are board-
certified but if they've completed the proper course
requirements, and if they're still active members (and if they
have sanctions against them).

4. Call your local hospital, which will have board-
certified plastic surgeons on staff. They won't allow
non-board-certified practitioners to do surgery because of the
malpractice risk, so they represent a good clearinghouse for
area surgeons.

So now you find yourself in the office of a plastic surgeon. How do you know what's important in helping you to choose him or not? First, at the initial consult, you may not even be talking with the surgeon—a nurse or assistant might be explaining the procedure to you. While that doesn't mean the surgeon isn't good, I believe that there's a level of patient-doctor rapport that cannot be fostered if the doctor's encounter with you is in the OR and no place else.

Assuming you're sitting across from the surgeon, ask these questions:

1. *Where do you have privileges?*

    It's good if it's at a prestigious hospital. (If it's not, however, and the surgeon is relatively young, that shouldn't be an automatic strike against. It takes time to get privileges.)

    If they don't have privileges at *any* nearby hospital, however, you should leave. Why? Because for their office to be accredited, they must have staff privileges at a local hospital. Therefore, without such privileges, their office is not accredited (which means the quality of care, the instrumentation, and the monitoring may not be as good).

    Don't take their word about hospital affiliation. Call the hospital to confirm that they're on staff where they say they are. During a recent malpractice trial, it came out that a New York surgeon's claims of hospital privileges were fabricated.

2. *How many times have you done this procedure?*

    If he says he's done two thousand face-lifts, look at him. Is he old enough for that to be true? It's fair to assume that many surgeons, both old and young, inflate their numbers a bit, since calculating exactly requires effort.

3. *Do you do your own follow-up?*

   When the operation is over, will you be seeing him or her, or an aide? Although it's not necessary for a surgeon to see you during follow-up, it's good medicine if we do.

4. *Who covers for you?*

   Is it their clinic? The local hospital? Another plastic surgeon? Is there a specific name they can give you? I know of a plastic surgeon who had an oral surgeon cover, postoperatively for his patients' postoperative tummy tuck. I'm not surprised that the oral surgeon didn't recognize a significant abdominal infection.

5. *What are the pre-op and post-op regimens, the limitations and risks?*

   A reputable plastic surgeon will explain all these to you. (Ask for it in writing because you'll forget.) Does he tell you about the limitations—for example, that a thighplasty won't remove every wrinkle but will only make your legs partially smoother? Does he explain the potential risks? Do you understand them?

6. *What kind of scars will I be left with?*

   Breast reduction leaves scars. A buttock lift leaves a large scar. Virtually every operation leaves a scar. The question to have answered is, how visible is the scar or scars? Understand where they will be, how big, and how wide they can become over time.

   (For African-Americans: Because of your greater risk of keloid scars—elevated, thick, hard scars that result from excess formation of collagen or scar tissue—particularly around the ears, ask the surgeon how he minimizes the risk. I find it helpful to alter my incisions slightly so they're not quite up against the ear, and to make sure there's no tension on the closure for both face-lifts and surgery around the nose.)

7. *Is this procedure the best and only one for achieving my goal?*

   To combat droopy lids, one doctor may suggest an upper-eyelid lift, where an eyebrow lift will achieve the better and longer-lasting effect. Once you've discussed what you want to fix, ask for the various options (if any) to achieve that effect, and the varying levels of success, risk, and price.

8. *What sort of anesthesia is used? Who gives it?*

   You can't be a surgeon and also administer unconscious anesthesia at the same time. You should have present in the OR either an anesthesiologist or a nurse-anesthetist. I'm partial to anesthesiologists because I think they have more training. But there are good nurse-anesthetists. Either way, there should be someone besides the surgeon in the OR who monitors the patient.

   If you suffer from a chronic condition such as diabetes, heart disease, or an autoimmune disease, it's smart to have the surgeon or anesthesiologist call your internist before your operation.

9. *Are you going away anytime soon?*

   You don't want to get surgery the day before he goes away for two weeks.

10. *How many operations do you do in a day, and what type?*

    Some surgeons do lots of operations in a day—six or seven noses, or four or five face-lifts, say—and it's tough to do a great job at that speed, and certainly impossible to put in every stitch yourself, meaning he's leaving the room and having an assistant (resident, nurse, or physician's assistant) close up his patients. I do every stitch myself not only because that's what I was taught to do but because complications are more easily avoided. It also means there will always be two physicians in the OR (the surgeon and the anesthesiologist). I do an average of twelve operations a week, not including Botox treatments and other quick fixes.

11. *Do you need to see old photos of me?* (This is particularly relevant for facial surgery.)

If he doesn't, then he's only seeing your face at one point in time—now—and won't have as educated a sense of your face's innate qualities (e.g., are your heavy lids the result of aging, or have you always had heavy upper lids?). This could affect the quality of your result. You may end up looking younger but less like yourself than you want.

The answers to the questions above, and the way in which the surgeon answers them, should go a good way in helping you to determine your comfort level. One question I recommend that patients *not* ask is *What do* you *think should be fixed?* What he thinks you need may not be what *you* think you need, and you may be offended to hear it. You need to know exactly what's made you unhappy enough to be there in the first place, tell the doctor what it is, then ask him what he thinks he can do about it.

Finally, during the consult, did the surgeon bad-mouth other doctors? If he did, be wary. While it's fine and appropriate, in my opinion, for the surgeon to say something negative about another doctor if it concerns an egregious breach of medical conduct, if he is more generally and excessively critical of doctors, then he may have an inflated sense of himself. This unrealistic frame of mind can make for a doctor with serious flaws.

A San Francisco patron of the arts had a surgeon remove a small, basal-cell skin cancer on her left upper lip. The good news? The cancer was cleared and she was cancer-free. The bad news? She neglected to choose a board-certified plastic surgeon (or didn't bother to ask him if he was certified, or didn't delve deeply enough to know it was even something to consider). The section of her upper lip he removed was replaced with a skin graft from her leg, which contracted within four months. (This case is now in litigation.)

For several months after that, she walked around with a perpetual snarl—or, rather, she was so devastated that she rarely left her house. Her gums were partly exposed; they dried out, causing erosion at the base of the tooth. Largely homebound and so embarrassed that she wore a surgical mask, she sought a friend's advice and found her way to my office. I removed the skin graft and started over, advancing her cheek skin into the upper lip. I followed a basic rule in (plastic) surgery: The best tissue match is almost always tissue immediately adjacent to the defect.

I closed the defect and she looked fine. Eight months later she returned to my office, no longer traumatized by plastic surgeons. "Now I'd like to have some surgery for my looks," she said. "A face-lift and a necklift."

"When were you thinking?" I asked.

"How's this afternoon?"

If he is honest, any self-respecting plastic surgeon will say he has never done a perfect job.

I've never done one, and, as a perfectionist, it haunts me. I lose sleep over work I've done. I run over in my mind how it could have been better. *Could I have removed more skin? Could I have put more cartilage in the nose?*

But if a patient is unhappy with the work I've done, I ask myself even more questions. *Did I make a technical error? Should I have operated in the first place? Was it the wrong procedure? Was it something about the patient?*

Sometimes you come up short for reasons beyond your control, influences such as the elasticity and pliability of skin, or the patient's history—smoking, or cocaine exposure to the nasal septum. Yet still I reassess the operation, my technique, and our pre-op analysis.

If you care about what you do, this taunt never goes away. It drives you to work harder, read journals, take more courses, attend more lectures, so you learn more and you improve, technically, to the point where you try slowly to innovate, coming up with better techniques than your peers'.

Learn, learn, learn.

Still, the result is never prefect.

Two Frenchmen in their forties came in, friends, both lawyers. Six months earlier, they had agreed to try a new synthetic filler reputed to work wonders at eliminating lines. A surgeon injected the filler, called Artecoll (approved in Europe but not yet in the United States), into the lines in their cheeks and their forehead wrinkles. Early results of the drug's effectiveness were encouraging, but that was from data collected over six months, hardly a long-term sample.

The two men paid the price. By the time they came to me, their faces were streaked red, with pus oozing from the holes where they'd been injected. They had tried to style their hair and use makeup as best they could to cover up their foreheads. It didn't matter. They looked ghoulish.

These men, who had been looking to take only a small step to improve their appearance, sat in my office distraught.

They'd already been through two rounds of antibiotics that hadn't worked. So I made small incisions around the infected sites, cut out the filler, and closed it up with fine sutures to minimize the scarring. I used nylon stitches, which are less likely to cause a reaction than the equally common synthetic sutures or sutures made of sheep's intestines. There was minor scarring.

The lesson to be learned: Before you take any new drug or undergo any new procedure, wait at least one full year after it's been on the market—especially if it's elective surgery!

It's impossible to avert failure all the time. The best I could do was minimize its chances. To help me, I kept a list of those things that all successful plastic surgeons do.

- Know your field but never forget what the competition is up to (through journals, conversation, conferences).
- Listen to your patients.
- Have an accredited office.
- Operate smoothly, quickly, decisively, carefully.
- Plan your surgery.
- Anticipate what can go wrong and plan to avoid it.
- Work nights and weekends.
- Be patient and diplomatic.
- Affiliate with an academic program.
- Diversify the range of procedures you do . . . but not too much.
- Stay humble. Solicit help from colleagues, former mentors, and patients.
- Remember always: Your first wife is surgery.

She Dies,
You Die:
The Royal Treatment
▼ ▼ ▼

She was my first European royal.

The day before she showed up for the consultation, her security detail came to check out my office.

Are the windows bulletproof?

Who's next door to your office, and what kind of access do they have?

There'd been occasions when the bodyguards and security for other royals or members of the Forbes 400 had checked me out—doing background workups without my knowledge, even following me—to confirm that I was competent and discreet. Yet this was the first time my office had been inspected.

Although my windows were not bulletproof, the bodyguards seemed satisfied. But now they had *me* worried. If the princess showed up for the consultation with two bodyguards, I wondered if we shouldn't be meeting not in my personal office, which had a window, but deeper inside my warren of rooms, such as my exam room, which had no window. Was there really someone out there who wanted to harm this lovely woman, as one of the security agents had suggested? What about a bomb?

The princess, blond and petite, turned out to be as gracious and easygoing as her handlers were not. It was one of the easiest preps and post-ops I'd ever had. The face-lift was a success. Everything worked out fine, despite my expecting complications and having nagging thoughts about an assassination attempt that might take me out as well.

Come to think of it, I was kind of glad to see her go.

For a Park Avenue plastic surgeon, socializing with successful people is a professional necessity. Not everyone I work on owns a jet, but lots of them do—usually a DeHavilland or a Gulfstream V. I want every patient on whom I perform a face-lift or chin implant or tummy tuck, etc., to love the results, and I work on everyone with an equal amount of care. But there are patients—the famous and the influential—who had *really* better love their results.

When a powerful, socially prominent person recommends you, it can translate into more patients and referrals—lots of them. Conversely, a bad word from a dissatisfied, tastemaking patient can do enormous damage to your practice, even destroy it. My colleagues and I tend to lose far more sleep over a well-known news anchor or actress or Manhattanite unhappy with her eyebrow lift than we do over a malpractice suit. (For one, lawsuits are an occupational hazard and happen to us all; for another, I've never lost one.)

These type-A people are more finicky, too. The ones from New York and L.A. are my most particular (more so than those from other parts of the country and from outside the United States). If I tell them they should get Botox every five months, you can be sure that, when their session is complete, they go right to Tanya and schedule an appointment for exactly five months later. And they're more demanding: If I say I'm booked for eight weeks, they insist that that can't be. They try to work my office manager.

In short, if you want to succeed as a Park Avenue surgeon, you are *always* on call. Your social life is an extension of your professional life; the main difference is that you're not wearing scrubs.

You'd better own a good tuxedo and know the right way to hold the stem of a flute. You'd better have a decent grasp of what's going on with geopolitical conflict and trade policy. You'd be well-served to speak, or at least know several phrases in, something other than just English (I know French fluently, and enough German, Italian, Spanish, Turkish, and Japanese to get by). You'd better attend parties, be gregarious, serve on the board of prestigious museums, and make it to charity functions.

Worldly people are interesting, diverse, and fun to be around. You want to be their friends because they improve the quality of your life. But sometimes they become more than just an operation.

Sometimes, a lot more.

I agreed to do a face-lift, eyelidplasty, and rhinoplasty for a queen and her lady-in-waiting. Months before, one of her representatives had begun to investigate me, unbeknownst to me. It was never clear what exactly Mohammed Ibraham's title was; "ambassador without portfolio," he called himself. An attractive, impeccably groomed man dressed in fine English suits with French cuffs, Mohammed spoke several languages with a true accent. He could charm the pants off a dictator. Occasionally, we would bump into each other at a cocktail party. He included me at state dinners. He was immensely likable. I just thought he was one of those fascinating people you meet in New York, Gstaad, London, or Hong Kong.

After several months he said, "I would like you to meet Her Majesty." He declined to say which country she was majesty of, though I had my suspicions. I thought it was just a social encounter— an honor, of course, but that was it. When she and Mohammed appeared one day at my office, I remembered to bow low. And to be polite. It quickly became clear that she and I could communicate neither in English nor her primary language; she spoke Japanese, as well, so I used the little Japanese I'd studied in college. She was trim and smartly dressed in Western-style clothes. She had a dark complexion, beautifully shaped brown eyes, and long lashes. She'd had acne as a child, so there was some facial scarring. Her smile was quick.

After a few pleasantries she quizzed me.

"Do you do face work?"

"Yes," I said.

"Can you do my eyes?"

"Yes."

After ten minutes she seemed satisfied. "I would like you to do it tomorrow morning."

I was floored. "That's not possible," I told her. "There's lab work to be—"

There was a knock on the door. I walked over and opened it. Mohammed stood there, a folder in his hand. I looked at it. All the queen's labs had been done—blood test, EKG, stress, everything.

"Well," I said, "it's not so easy. I'd have to move a lot of things around . . ."

Mohammed shot me an expression that said, *Be real.* I'd had experience with movie stars and wealthy South Americans expecting to be fit in quickly, but this took the cake.

I called the head of OR at one of the hospitals I'm affiliated with, and asked what the odds were of getting a room the next day—no, make that *two* ORs, which Her Majesty required for the privacy and comfort of her bodyguards. Before he could object, I said, "It's a queen. Of a country. Money is no object."

All of a sudden, doors opened up. I called the chief of anesthesiology and got what I needed.

The next day, the queen was wheeled into the operating room followed by the chief of the king's security detail, assigned to the queen. Heavily built, hair slicked back, five foot six on tiptoes, Ali's professional style was as hostile to the concept of "subtlety" as mine was measured by it. When he smiled, I could see every crooked tooth. He had a gun. In a shoulder strap. In his sterile gown and coverings and surgical mask and cap, his bulk looked almost absurd.

I scrubbed. The anesthesiologist stood there, waiting. As I readied to be gowned and gloved, Ali offered the most memorable vote of confidence I've ever heard.

"If she dies," he said in heavily accented English to my anesthesiologist, and I could tell by the crinkles around his eyes that he was smiling his crooked-toothed smile under the mask, "I will kill the doctor and you."

The anesthesiologist stared at him.

"I have diplomatic immunity," he said.

The anesthesiologist, shaking, turned to me. "Does he?"

"Yes," I said.

Excitement, international people...it's not as if my out-of-the-OR life didn't have its moments.

While at a fund-raiser for the Conservation Committee at the Museum of the City of New York, I was seated next to Sarah Ferguson, Duchess of York—Fergie—and her lady-in-waiting. We danced, we talked, we laughed; she was funny and vibrant and amazingly chipper for someone who'd once undergone worldwide scrutiny and humiliation, from a toe-sucking to divorce to public ouster from a certain family in England. Good for her not to allow her natural effusiveness to get beaten out of her.

Unless I was mistaken, she was making a pass at me. "So what are you doing next week?" she purred, leaning over the table and smiling.

Stunned, I didn't reply.

"We're going to India," said Fergie, gesturing at her lady-in-waiting to show that there would be a chaperone. "Would you like to come along?"

I'm sure I turned some shade of beet.

"I have to work," I stammered, an unfortunate excuse.

I was invited to a formal reception at the French ambassador's residence on Park Avenue in honor of Louis de Bourbon, a member of French royalty. The walls were covered with Matisses, Manets, and paintings on loan from the Louvre. There were ambassadors from Europe, Africa, and the Middle East, all chatting and laughing with each other. The Russian and French contingents parried over which nation really had a better understanding of fascism, while the Moroccan ambassador and the U.N. representative from Spain playfully jabbed at each other. The Moroccan said that Spain should return the three towns it occupied that rightfully belonged to Morocco.

"We'll give them back," said the U.N. rep, "when you get the British to return Gibraltar to us."

Just before dinner, a commotion broke out across the room. Two gorgeous women in their midforties, in ballgowns, were slapping at each other.

"Bitch!" one yelled.

"Screw you!" the other said.

Then they really started clawing.

The rest of the room—mostly men—stood and watched. No one did anything. A roomful of diplomats and experts in international relations, and no one wanted to get involved. Which side to choose?

As the only person there not involved in diplomacy, I grabbed each woman by an arm and separated them. But then I thought, *What do I do now?* They were still fighting. The first order of business was to get them outside. I led them down the long, winding staircase, as they continued swearing and swinging at each other.

We walked out onto Park Avenue.

It was freezing. They were in their ballgowns, me in my tuxedo.

I hoped a cooling of body temperature would have the desired effect on their systems. The ladies continued yelling at each other, but they had given up on taking swings, preferring to use their arms to keep themselves warm. Still, they continued the verbal attacks.

"Bitch," one of them said halfheartedly, shivering.

The other one, hugging herself, didn't bother to reply.

After another moment, I finally asked them what had happened.

The lady in the yellow ballgown, the wife of an ambassador, accused the lady in the pale blue ballgown, the girlfriend of another ambassador, of having stiffed her dressmaker.

I nodded. We walked around the block. I admonished them for embarrassing themselves and their partners. But even more bothersome is that we had embarrassed our gracious host. How, we all wondered, could we possibly return? We needed an excuse to re-enter the party. They looked to me. I said that I wasn't sure what we would say, but I would figure something out by the time we returned.

As we walked up the stairs, thoughts raced through my mind. As we turned the corner to the dining area, it was like a scene from a movie: Fifty couples in black tie and formal gowns, surrounded by servants, all stopped their conversation to stare at us.

The three of us stood there.

I said the only thing I could think of: "It's amazing what people will do to get a consult. And I'm *not* going to tell you what part of their bodies they asked about."

Everyone laughed. I got a kiss on each cheek. The party resumed.

▼

It was late afternoon. I had finished surgery for the day; Park Avenue seemed quiet. Across the street, Le Cirque had been turned, for several days, into a meeting place for peace talks between the Israelis and the Palestinians. The police had closed the street to cars, so the usual white noise of New York traffic outside my office was notable for its absence.

I was standing in my reception area, in scrubs, checking charts, when the door opened. Two Middle Eastern men walked in.

Yasser Arafat and his bodyguard.

I can't say I knew how to react. Arafat looked at me, sizing me up and down. He broke into a huge grin.

"I clearly have the wrong place," he said in heavily accented English.

He did not move. His eyes now slowly scanned the office—the waiting room, the stack of shelter and fashion magazines, perhaps the business cards on the desk that identified me as a plastic surgeon. He looked as scruffy as he did in photographs.

"But maybe I have the right place," he said, smiling.

I smiled and shrugged. He apologized, turned, and the two men left to find the right place.

I was invited to attend the horse races at Ascot, outside London, and had the privilege of meeting Princess Diana at a prerace reception. At the time, Diana was still with Charles. As I waited my turn to greet the princess, I thought fondly of my most vivid memory of her—watching her fairy-tale wedding on a TV over the bed of one of the patients in the cardiac care unit at Stanford University Hospital, taking in this vision of loveliness while, in my blood-spattered scrubs, I checked on the sick and dying. Seeing her now, in person,

I couldn't keep my eyes off her. She wore a navy suit and an Ascot-worthy hat, and she was inarguably attractive. But she was not what you'd call beautiful. From a strictly anatomical point of view, many women are more "perfect" than she.

Yet she radiated something. She had great skin. There was a slight heaviness to her eyebrows and upper lids, giving her a sultry air. Her eyes were clear blue and beautiful. Her smile was quick and genuine.

When finally it was my turn to meet her, her aide introduced me as "Dr. Cap Lesesne, plastic surgeon, from New York"—and before the last syllables were even out of his mouth, Princess Diana had lowered her gaze knowingly.

"Oh, really?" she said, smiling. "Well, we won't have anything further to say to you, will we?"

A Little Romance

▼ ▼ ▼

My practice was humming along, quietly getting attention at cocktail parties and dinners and even opening night at the opera. Because of what we do, we're never going to get a grateful actor or extremely satisfied diplomat to mention our skills and excellent results in a magazine profile—as a great chef or interior decorator might enjoy—the day after which your phone would be ringing off the hook. No, the right kind of attention for a Park Avenue plastic surgeon means this: Satisfied patients in the "discreet" professions—banking, law, international diplomacy, medicine—start whispering to their coworkers and friends that you're Their Guy. That doesn't mean I didn't want Hollywood people or politicians; of course I did. But the foundation for a great New York practice is to quietly expand beyond just the Upper East Side, whose reach in New York City affairs may be extensive and profound, but still has its limits.

Still, much social life and professional opportunity commingled, often on the Upper East Side. At a dinner party, I was seated next to Stephanie, the recently separated wife of one of the most powerful, visible men in the world (neither American nor European). She was attractive, intelligent, well-traveled, and likable, distracting me so that I ignored my partner to the left. Stephanie was in her late fifties, with four grown children. Ten minutes into our conversation she found an opening to say, "My husband left me for a younger woman."

"It makes no sense to you," I said, shaking my head, "and frankly, it makes no sense to me. He must have gone off the deep end."

"I don't understand it," she said, expressing confusion, even longing.

When Stephanie heard what I did, we talked about it for a while, but I thought, *She'd be difficult. To my eye she's beautiful, and if I did a classic lift, she'd lose some of her sex appeal. She would become too sculpted in the eyes, too sharp in the jawline. Little things would be better but something bigger would be lost.*

Her boyfriend came by. He was maybe fifteen years older than she, and graying. Five seconds after meeting him it was clear that he wasn't in her league. Not sharp enough, not elegant enough.

This woman can do so much better than him, I thought.

Before the end of dinner, she asked for my card. "Don't put it on the table," she said.

I reached under the table and placed my card on Stephanie's skirt.

One lady friend, after several dates, leaned over a candelit table in a restaurant and announced that she'd had her breasts done—something I was able to tell as soon as I'd hugged her. I couldn't help myself. "When were you going to mention the work you've had on your ears and your jaw?" I asked.

Sometimes I just couldn't shut off my PSR (Plastic Surgeon's Radar). Walking down the street or sitting at a reception, I automatically evaluated every person over forty. *Yes? No?* I could make out scarring that others might miss. I checked out the shape of the earlobes to see if they'd been slightly altered from what you'd expect. I might sneak a peek at the base of their nose, where some surgeons hide their scars. It was my disease.

Another woman I dated, a magazine editor I liked and admired, insisted that I never tell her what work she might benefit from (I didn't, nor was I planning to). Then, at a Thanksgiving dinner, she kept needling me in front of others about how I continually refused to tell her what she needed. "Cap keeps that info to himself," she said.

I'm doing nothing of the sort, I thought. Since we'd met weeks before, my PSR had *not* been "on" with her, nor was it on that night. I thought she was attractive and I liked her. Period.

But she badgered me throughout the evening. I just shook my head to let others know it wasn't true.

"Look," she said. "He's looking at me like he's figuring out what to do first."

Finally, unable to stop her taunting (though she was really taunting herself), I'd had it. I switched on my PSR, full bore.

When she went to the kitchen, I followed her. From the oven she pulled an overcooked turkey.

"Here," she said, handing me a dull knife. "You're the surgeon. Cut the bird."

It was impossible to slice the dry turkey. It just crumbled. I needed a better knife, but she crossed her arms, disappointed in my skills.

I looked in her eyes and blurted, "You'd be so much more beautiful with a smaller nose."

She grabbed the knife from me. "Bastard!" she shouted, and started stabbing at the turkey. It was the beginning of the end of our relationship.

Some clients were *too* pleased with my work.

Naomi, a Stanford MBA in her forties, divorced mother of one son, was delighted by the necklift I'd performed on her; she'd had quite a bit of excess skin and now it was smooth. When she showed up for her follow-up, she was very friendly. On her second follow-up, she brought homemade cookies, as well as a CD of arias, because she knew from casual conversation that I like opera. Then she leaned forward.

"I had a fantasy," she said, smiling slyly at me. "You were in it."

As a doctor, you walk a fine line. You need to say the right thing to maintain professionalism, yet you can't come off as cold.

I just smiled.

"Not a dream fantasy," she continued. "A waking one. Let's take a trip to Europe. Go to art museums. The Pergamon, the Rijksmuseum."

I chuckled. For once, I didn't know what to say.

She called the office a couple times the next week. I just hoped her infatuation would run its course, or that she would get the idea.

At another reception, I waited on the buffet line to get dinner—and there she was: Stephanie, the charming woman I'd sat next to at another dinner party, whose powerful and famous husband had left her for a younger woman.

Stephanie looked great. She hadn't had any cosmetic surgery done in the meantime.

"I'd like you to meet my husband," she said, and tugged on the hand of the man whose back was to her.

It was the boyfriend. The older man who couldn't hold a candle to her.

It lasted for only a moment, but I caught a sadness in Stephanie's eyes.

At times it's unbearable to think that, simply because of how aging manifests physically, women, in particular, are less and less seen and appreciated for who they are—their character, their accomplishments, their sexiness. Way too often, others don't see it. They themselves don't see it. And so they settle for less than they deserve.

▼

Naomi, the grateful necklift patient who seemed to like me, one day appeared in my office just before noon, wondering if she could take me to lunch. I had to decline, politely.

She was starting to creep me out.

Walking briskly down Madison Avenue at five thirty in the morning on my way to the office, I had stopped for the light at Seventieth Street when I heard a crash. I turned to see that the plate-glass window of the Italian shoestore on the corner had shattered, and a man was emerging from the store holding a cashbox. From not ten feet away, he looked at me, and I at him, and we seemed equally startled and puzzled by each other. Then it dawned on me that he'd just that moment finished robbing the store—or, it dawned further, that he'd just finished the robbing part and had yet to begin the getaway, which was about to commence. With no help from my conscious mind, I automatically scanned him, from the top of his LA baseball cap down to his tan Timberland work boots. *Navy blue parka, blue jeans. Five feet ten, 180 pounds. Mole, two centimeters from left nostril. Crooked upper-front two teeth. Brown eyes, slightly graying hair on side of cap. Pimple on upper right cheek. Attached earlobes.*

"Call the police," he said, staring straight at me. "There's someone hurt inside."

And he took off down the block.

It was brilliant of him, I would later think. In that shared frozen moment, our minds had both been racing, doing the things we were trained to do: I, the surgeon, spent it gathering data about his face and physique that might be useful; he, the thief, spent it scrambling for a way to best immobilize the bystander before him, so that he could make a successful getaway.

As soon as I stepped inside the store, I realized it for the lie it was: No one was there, hurt or otherwise. Back outside, I spotted his retreating figure a half block away, running for Central Park. Again, not thinking, I gave chase. The adrenaline rush was similar to what you feel when you're trying to save a life. As I ran past a residential building, I yelled at the doorman—sleeping in a chair just inside the entrance, his cap tipped down over his eyes—to call 911. Continuing west, I saw the thief enter the park, then lost sight of him. At the park entrance, I scanned the area in front of me, but he was gone. Out of breath, I returned to the building where I'd yelled to the doorman, took the phone from him, and gave the police a detailed description. Then I ran to the park. Within a minute, a squad car appeared a couple blocks south of me and I ran into the street, hopping up and down, yelling and waving. He floored it in reverse and pulled up alongside me. Without hesitating I jumped in the backseat and told them I was the one who'd seen the robber. The cop in the front passenger seat said they'd already called in to have the park sealed, and the lights turned on, a show of authority that mightily impressed me. As we passed through a break in the park wall at Sixty-ninth Street, I began rattling off the description again.

"LA baseball cap, navy blue parka, blue jeans. Five-ten, one-eighty, mole two centimeters from left nostril. Crooked upper-front two teeth. Pimple on upper right cheek—"

The cop in the passenger seat shifted full around to look at me. "Who the fuck are you?"

I didn't understand what he meant.

"I never heard a description like this," he said.

"Oh. I'm a plastic surgeon."

"Shit," he said, shaking his head. "I never heard a description like that."

Five minutes later, about six fifteen now, a call came through that another patrol car cruising the park had stopped someone matching my description. The robber had done himself in: The cops had noticed a man jogging, in parka, blue jeans, and heavy work boots. When they stopped him for questioning, he said he was out jogging. In parka, jeans, and work boots.

It came out that he'd been arrested thirty times. He was convicted, got fifteen years. After the trial, the DA told me he'd never heard a description like that.

It was after business hours. I opened the door to leave my office, and right away I knew someone was lurking in the hallway who didn't belong there.

I was pushed back against the wall.

Then she tried to kiss me.

Naomi had been lying in wait. She had seen the lights go out. Before I knew what was going on, she'd pushed me back inside my office and her face was pressed up to mine.

I admit it: I was scared. Plastic surgeons have stalkers who occasionally carry guns. One doctor in Seattle was shot.

I knew the cleaning lady was in one of the rooms.

"Gloria!" I yelled—not for her help, but so my psycho patient would know we were not alone.

"Doctor, I want you," said Naomi.

"Gloria!" I yelled again. "Naomi, I do not date patients," I said quietly. *"Gloria!"*

The door to my inner office opened, and Gloria appeared.

Naomi unclenched me and ran from the office.

I met a fun, supportive, pretty woman. She worked as a paralegal at a big matrimonial law firm. She'd been married twice before. She had two children.

Her name was Elsie.

It had been so long that my mind was one-track about surgery that it wouldn't have been startling had I simply *forgotten* to seek more permanent companionship and the promise of a family.

After dating me steadily for some time, Elsie said, "If you don't propose, I'm leaving."

I probably should have told her, *No, this isn't going to work out.*

Should have cut my losses right there.

But I said nothing.

She had called so many times in the two weeks before her face-lift—wanting to re-re-review the procedure, wanting the fee reduced, *This is a problem, that's a problem*—that I should just have told her, *I'm sorry, but you'll have to find someone else to do this.*

I said nothing.

I performed the operation. Jiang Li looked sensational. Her daughter agreed that her mother looked sensational. But that meant nothing to Jiang Li. She was unhappy—with the face-lift, with me, with her daughter, with fluorescent light, with herself, with life. She had been a famous singer in China, and she could not get over the fact that she was no longer desired, no longer beautiful as she defined beautiful—the complex beauty of a forty-seven-year-old, the full-throated beauty of a thirty-five-year-old, the gossamer beauty of a twenty-three-year-old. She was sixty-two. She had moments, you could tell, where she believed she still had fame and accomplishment and music in her. But then she would look in the mirror, and whoever it was who looked back did not agree.

A month later, she was admitted to a psychiatric home.

Not that it would have mattered, but I should have said no.

▼

If the romantic intensity and spontaneity of the proposal are indicative of the chance for marital success, then we were doomed from the start.

In response to Elsie's ultimatum ("If you don't propose, I'm leaving"), I had thought for maybe a few seconds, then said, "Will you marry me?"

Not six months into the marriage, my relationship with Elsie started to crumble. We fought sporadically, then regularly. There were too many times, for my liking, when I wasn't home and alcohol was involved, that the police came to the house.

Finally, we separated. One day, Elsie called to ask if I'd drive with her through a snowstorm to deliver something to her daughter. I had the flu but I agreed. After we finished the errand, I returned with Elsie to the house where she was living, and went to collapse in an upstairs bedroom. But soon I heard crashing noises coming from below. I walked down the stairs—and just as I reached the landing, a bottle flew past my head, missing me by inches and shattering against the wall behind me.

I looked over to see Elsie, at the bar, reaching for another liquor bottle. Before she could snatch it, I moved quickly toward her and grabbed her arm. In an effort to cool the situation down, I pushed her out the door.

I called the police to report it. When the cops came, they asked what happened, and when I recounted how I'd pushed Elsie out the door, they shook their heads. As soon as I had put my hands on her and removed her from the premises—though she had thrown a bottle at my head—I had committed third-degree assault, a misdemeanor. I was arrested.

Elsie dropped the charges.

But prospects for our marriage dropped faster.

After splitting up, we remained friendly, for a while. We were out of each other's lives cleanly and abruptly. We hadn't had any children together. We weren't involved long enough for her children and me to form deep bonds. She and I had lived under the same roof for less than two years.

Except for the possibility that every now and then we might cross paths in Manhattan, the biggest little small town, I expected that, compared to most ex-spouses, we would fade faster and more completely from each other's view, and that would be that.

The Royal Treatment, Part II

▼ ▼ ▼

My erudite, multinational friend Mohammed, the man who had introduced me to Her Royal Majesty, was on the phone.

"The queen would like you to come visit," Mohammed said warmly. She wished to have more work done, he told me, and several of her companions wished it, too. I told him I would have a little free time in a month, when I would be halfway to her part of the world, taking a long weekend in the south of France.

"Fine," he said. "The plane will pick you up there when you have concluded your stay."

Mohammed would not tell me what work was to be done, so when the date approached, I would have to messenger over to his office an extensive set of instruments and injectables, to be prepared for anything. It was all very James Bondian.

A month later, I stood in my tuxedo on the porch of the Hôtel de Paris in Monte Carlo, sipping Moët and watching fireworks explode over the harbor. Roger Moore, 007 himself, stood just feet away, looking even more dashing than he does on-screen. In another corner were Arnold Scaasi, Joan Collins, and Veruschka. We'd all been invited to help celebrate the twenty-fifth wedding anniversary of our friends Ricky and Sandra di Portanova of Houston and Acapulco, legends in the international jet set. The party was so glamorous that celebrities from a nearby event—Jerry Lee Lewis, Marlo Thomas, and the CEOs of FedEx and Northwest Airlines, to name a few—joined us. Assessing the scene all around me, I was truly amid the glitterati—and it wasn't the champagne talking: I'd had the bartender cut it with seltzer six times because there was a chance I'd have to operate the next day. The queen's people were flying me to her country the following morning. Given the veil of secrecy surrounding my work on her, who knew? I might be asked to operate immediately upon my arrival. Mohammed, as usual, had been sparse with details. I'd been told only that I would be gone for four to five days. I did not know where I was being taken—the Middle East, Southeast Asia, or someplace completely different.

Here in Monte Carlo, though, in the summer of 1999, on the porch of the elegant Hôtel de Paris, having a ball, smiling and chitchatting, everything seemed like a fairy tale, something out of *To Catch a Thief;* I almost expected Cary Grant and Grace Kelly to appear on a nearby balcony. I watched Veruschka hit on the younger guys. The once-beautiful Slavic was lean and still striking, but her skin was sun-ravaged. She reminded me of Brigitte Bardot; aging, I thought, is a relentless and indiscriminate bully. Joan Collins was on a couch teasing Arnold Scaasi; she, on the other hand, had aged well and had had good work. And wore her makeup well.

What a surreal scene. Maybe my focus on work really was unhealthy, I thought. The demands of my job meant I was in the office by seven, almost always in bed by ten. I had to keep my emotions in check. I hardly drank. I didn't even play golf.

These people, though: Man, they knew how to live.

I'd become friends with the di Portanovas, our hosts, through Jeanette Longoria, a patient many times over and now a close friend. A Texan, Ricky di Portnova was descended on his father's side from Italian royalty, and on his mother's from an oil fortune, one of the largest privately held oil developers in the world. Back in the sixties, though, Ricky had been a sculptor, moved to Rome, married a Yugoslavian basketball player, and lived a bohemian life. He fell out of touch with his family back home and eventually concluded that he'd been disinherited.

One morning, he was awakened by a knock on his door. Standing there were two Houston lawyers who informed him that he'd been named in his grandfather's will, and that he might want to return home. Some money was involved. Three million dollars.

Tax-free.

Each month.

In perpetuity.

Stateside, Ricky's marriage to the Yugoslav disintegrated. One day, the newly minted multimillionaire walked into a soda shop in Austin, Texas. His eyes met those of an undergrad behind the counter, a young woman of Armenian descent named Sandra Hovar. Lost to history is what Ricky ordered from her. Not lost is the fact that Sandy, nicknamed Buckets because of her beautiful breasts, leaned over to serve him.

Ricky fell in.

Oh, he told himself, *that's what I want.*

Soon enough, Sandy became Princess di Portanova, with homes in Houston, Acapulco, and London. When she shopped internationally, she sometimes took along a second 737 to lug everything home.

Now, looking out at the Monte Carlo harbor and marveling at the spectacular light show of the international fireworks festival that lit up the summer sky, I sipped one more half-glass of watered-down champagne and called it a night.

Early in the morning, a car arrived to take me to the airport. I was instructed to go to a certain desk, where a ticket awaited me. No destination was printed on the ticket, nor was one listed on the marquee behind the desk. Passengers milled about.

My flight was called to board. I was first. Entering the 747 cabin, I looked to the right, into coach, to see . . . no one. Looking left, into business and first class, I saw . . . no one. The only people on the plane were the crew.

"Good morning, Dr. Lesesne, and welcome aboard," the steward said to me, ushering me to my first-class seat.

After several minutes, I realized I was the only passenger.

As we took off and the plane banked to the right, I watched from the window. I had no idea where I was being taken, and no control over it—a pretty tough thing for a surgeon to swallow—so I just let go.

I slept off and on. Once, I attempted to engage a flight attendant in a conversation about our destination. He smiled broadly and asked if I wished more food or drink.

I awoke as we began our descent, nine hours after leaving the ground. Looking out, I saw a gorgeous coastline rimming the aquamarine of the Pacific. Or was it the Indian Ocean? Now I could make out a lone airstrip. Other than that, nothing but sand and water as far as the eye could see. When the plane door opened, a blast of furnace-hot air hit me, tempered only slightly by the ocean breeze. I descended the steps. At the bottom, a familiar face greeted me.

It was Ali, the barrel-chested head of his country's security. The last time we had seen each other—at the OR at the hospital in New York, where I had done a face-lift on Her Majesty—Ali had told me that if the queen died, he would kill me.

"Masa'a Alkair," I said to him now. Since our last meeting, I had mastered a few Arabic phrases.

Ali grinned. "Dr. Lesesne, welcome," he said, holding out his hand. "May I please have your passport?"

I hesitated.

"You won't be needing it," he assured me. I handed it to him.

He took it, then held out his hand again. "And may I please have your wallet." Before I could hesitate, he said, "You won't be needing that, either."

He wasn't smiling. He took all my forms of identification.

Everything would be returned to me, Ali announced, after the surgeries. "You are a guest of His Majesty's government," he said.

Now he smiled.

One could interpret the gesture as intimidating. I chose to view it as the ultimate gesture of hospitality.

In a Spartan-looking building beside the airstrip, Saudis in beautiful, deep purple, gold-trimmed robes mingled with Russian oil executives. I was ushered into a black Mercedes, accompanied by Ali and a driver. For an hour we sped inland, through desert the color of faded bone. No more sightings of water; there was sand, sky, and nothing else. At the moment, I literally had no identity (no passport, no wallet) and was careening through a foreign country. I was putting a lot of trust in them, just as they had in me. Every now and then, sand swirled up from the desert. The dunes rose and fell like waves, like the contours of the body. I remembered the first time, as a young surgeon-to-be, that I'd incised skin, and how it was nothing at all like cutting into an animal, nothing like a cadaver. The sensation of the skin is mostly resistance—a reaction pressing back against the scalpel, the singular pressure that simply cannot be understood by reading medical textbooks; you must feel it. And then the first time you see bleeding. All the feedback that goes through your fingers to your brain. *I'm becoming a surgeon,* you think—and then you realize just how much you don't know. Outside the Mercedes, there were no signs of life, just two endless colors, the café au lait of desert, the undiluted azure of sky. You focus on what you are doing, you don't look up at the overseeing doctor across the table as he talks to you. You're so scared you feel as if you'll wet your pants. Early on, a mentor observes every cut, on every procedure. Then he's there less and less. A few years pass and suddenly you're no longer removing appendices or benign lipomas but standing over someone with complex facial fractures and you've got a high-speed drill in your hands and you're putting screws around their skull and moving their eyeballs around and if you sneeze you'll either blind them for life or kill them.

An amazing transformation.

I spotted my first goat, weighed down by his pack and led by an old man. Then more goats. Then crossroads, houses, and finally a sign.

At least I knew where I was.

We entered the city. I rolled down the window and smelled salt air again. The scenery turned greener and greener. In the distance, finally, I saw it: the castle, the color of wet cinnamon, with towers and square parapets at each end. Its perimeter was brocaded by palm and date trees—as well as security guys, soldiers, and police. Guns everywhere. We passed through the guard gate into a central square within the castle.

We got out of the car. "Your quarters are through here," said Ali, and I followed him across the sun-bleached square, inside the castle, and down many stone steps. Suddenly, we were outside again, and I was looking out on the most spectacular beach I had ever seen. Its beauty took my breath away. Its serenity would have, too, but every fifteen feet stood another sentry with a gun, from one of the country's three armed services.

"Dr. Lesesne?" Ali said, waving me on. "Your room is in the basement."

I was led down a dungeonlike passageway and then, to my shock, to a cramped, damp room. After all the top-notch travel and amenities, I was a little stunned.

"I can't believe you're putting me here," I said in a tone more confrontational than I'd meant. It had been a long day.

"The room does not please you?" he said.

"Honestly? It might be better for Your Majesty if I stayed at a hotel."

Ali bowed his head. "That is fine."

Ten minutes later, as I entered the downtown Hyatt Regency flanked by Ali and another bodyguard, two gorgeous, familiar-looking native women, dressed in Chanel, passed us. One of them turned.

"Dr. Lesesne?" she said. "What are you doing here?"

Quickly noting my companions, she put two and two together, smiled, and walked on.

Thank you, I thought.

My security guys looked at me funny. "I did not believe you knew anybody here," said Ali.

"Dumb luck," I said. They were sisters I'd performed lipo on a month before, in New York.

Up in my hotel room, I was convinced the place was bugged. After all, these guys left nothing to chance. But it was a magical moment. I set down my bag, opened the window, and reveled in the present. I scanned the view of the minarets of the mosques, of the small houses and the people walking below. At that instant, in the hot, dusty twilight, the imams started their call for evening prayers. The air was filled with a scent of flowers, animals, and the sweet fruit in the stalls below.

I gazed out the window for a long time. I reflected on how, when I was training to be a surgeon, never did I imagine that I would find myself in such a place or such a moment. Yet here I was, experiencing exactly the kind of life I'd dreamed of as a young boy. Only I'd made it here not as an international lawyer but as a doctor.

I was a long, long way from Grosse Pointe.

I walked back to the bed, lay down, and drifted off into a wonderful, secure sleep.

An hour later, the telephone rang. Ali was calling from the lobby.

"Doctor, come down. We're ready to go."

Outside the hotel, yet another black car awaited me. This one was flanked by two men, both with handguns. I was whisked to yet another oceanside vacation estate, this one owned by my new friend Ali. A wedding was going on. The country's entire cabinet was there, along with regional dignitaries. Many of the women wore Western dress, but some, their hands painted in oil, danced in traditional folk dress. I watched the scene, fascinated.

Ali turned to me. "Is there anything you would like to do while you are here?"

"I'd like to see the most beautiful mosques," I said.

Everyone within earshot turned. Ali and the rest smiled at me, but perplexed smiles.

"Why?" asked Ali. "You're an American. You're not Muslim."

"I've seen pictures and so many of them are breathtaking. I'm interested in mosques."

Again they smiled, perplexed. "I belong to a group in New York called Friends of Islamic Art," I said.

"A political group?" one asked.

"The Metropolitan Museum of Art," I said.

Their smiles lit up the room.

Finally, I could let go a little bit. I allowed myself to drink several different wines, but just a few sips of each. I had no idea what tomorrow would bring.

Early the next morning there was a knock on my door. I was driven to the castle, where, finally, I got to do what I'd been summoned for. The queen, the wife of the army chief, and Ali's wife, along with all their several ladies-in-waiting, got dermabrasion, collagen, and Botox. No one demanded anything taxing. (No anesthesia was required.) Everything went smoothly.

Now all I had to do was wait two or three days while Her Majesty recovered.

The results, I knew, had better be good.

In the days waiting for the ladies to heal, I was escorted to visit the mosques—their glittering domes, the white walls and minarets, the phenomenal views they offered of desert and sea. I explored the surrounding countryside and ate every single meal under the watchful eyes of Ali, the chief of police, and numerous bodyguards. It's hard to imagine warmer, more gracious hosts. It's hard to imagine that—God forbid something went awry with one of the royal procedures—they would actually have killed me.

Finally, after checking in with Her Majesty and her ladies once more, it was agreed by all that, yes, the work was more than satisfactory.

Maybe we would meet next time in New York.

"*Inshallah,*" I said, their customary good-bye. *If God wills it.*

My passport and wallet were returned. I was flown first-class to New York. Months later, I received an invitation to the wedding of one of the royal daughters.

Since then, I have occasionally wondered why I wasn't more worried about the possibility—highly unlikely, of course, but within the realm—that something might go wrong.

But I never gave it a second thought.

Professionally, at least, I was as sure of myself as I could be.

Reconstruction

▼ ▼ ▼

L isa Gaylord, my OR nurse at the time, and I were driving to my Westchester office when traffic just stopped. We couldn't see what was happening, so I pulled my car onto the shoulder, stepped out, and walked toward the commotion.

There had been a head-on collision a minute before.

In one car, an older man was unconscious and cut up, but he did not appear critically hurt. Two bystanders lifted him from his car and laid him on the road with his legs up, so he wouldn't go into shock. Shortly, he regained consciousness.

From the second car came the stink of burning rubber. The driver was slumped against the steering wheel. A volunteer fireman and I pulled him out.

The man, who looked about thirty, had no pulse. No respiration. He bled from the mouth. He was turning blue.

Brain damage begins within three minutes of total oxygen deprivation.

Lisa started giving him CPR and we got a heartbeat. But still no breathing. I tried to get air into him via mouth-to-mouth, but I couldn't form a seal. The man was turning bluer.

I would have to do a tracheotomy.

The only remotely surgical-like instrument Lisa and I had between us was a penknife. I cut into his swollen neck—or more accurately, I sawed into it, so dull was the knife blade—and cut down to the trachea, hoping I didn't hit his carotid artery; if I did, and if he really wasn't dead already, then he'd *absolutely* be dead. With my finger, I swept the muscles away, feeling the cartilage of his trachea against my index finger. I could now see it was the trachea. I cut out an H-shaped hole but still couldn't form a seal to breathe into it for resuscitation.

Fortunately, a police officer had arrived with an oxygen tank and, at least as important, tubing.

I cut a beveled edge at one end of the tube, slid that end into the trach hole, and we turned on the oxygen.

Seconds later, the man turned pink.

It's exhilarating to save a life, especially when you've witnessed so many lives that weren't savable.

I thought I was starting to get a sense of who I was, first and last—namely, that my destiny was to help others, which I loved doing more than anything, but perhaps at the price of my own domestic and romantic fulfillment.

That was okay. But, as a plastic surgeon, I bristled a little at the notion that what I did most of the time with my medical training was somehow less valuable than what I *might* be doing with it. It's the question that every plastic surgeon gets, and frequently.

"So, doing breastlifts and nosejobs and face-lifts and tummy tucks is probably satisfying, but they don't compare to what it feels like doing a facial reconstruction or helping a burn victim—right?"

Wrong.

I am not an ogre. I am not suggesting that doing facial reconstructive surgery, or helping to alleviate the effects of a childhood disease like cleft lip, or doing a skin graft on someone who's been in a fire, is not hugely gratifying. I am blessed and humbled that I have the ability to do this.

But all of it is equally gratifying, at least for me. And probably for most of my colleagues, too.

I became a plastic surgeon because I saw what it could do to change people's lives, to propel them to greater things. Simple as that. Yes, some changes and life results are bigger than others, but it can be presumptuous to decide whose life is more profoundly affected by one surgery or another. Doing a nosejob on someone who has always labored under the impression that she is ugly; removing saddlebags from a woman who has never walked past another human being, male or female, without obsessing that she is being looked at mockingly; enlarging the breasts of a woman who has never felt womanly; or removing jowly skin to restore a jawline to a man who believes his colleagues think he's over the hill . . . doing all that, so these people can feel more attractive, confident, desirable, better equipped to attract a man or a woman, or interview for a job, or just walk their dog on the beach . . . that's huge! Sure, you can argue it; you can say that it's all just elective surgery, after all; you can say that what's inside the person is still inside the person and you can't fundamentally change *that*. Having done thousands of elective surgeries that "merely" tweak and fix things on faces and bodies, I can tell you that what gets changed on the outside *can* alter the inside, despite what skeptics may think.

A provocative survey was recently done whose results I implicitly believe. A born optimist, the survey said, generally fights through tough times to retain his or her natural optimism, while a born pessimist, no matter the prosperity, eventually finds his or her way back to a pessimistic outlook. The study's most quotable example: An optimist who suffers an accident that leaves him quadriplegic will likely, after the shock and adjustment, eventually become an upbeat paraplegic, whereas a sourpuss who wins the lottery, after the thrill and adjustment, eventually becomes a grumpy millionaire. That doesn't work in all cases, of course, and there are many permutations and nuances to it. But I believe there's something inherently true about it.

Still, that doesn't mean that significant, life-altering transformations can't happen, because they do. I see it all the time, day after day, year after year, and it's my privilege to be part of and witness to them. For example, a fifty-year-old woman comes to me for Botox injections once every five months and now spends so much more time outdoors and socializing than she spends in her home, where she would often grow depressed and self-obsessed. Another example: the thirty-six-year-old who hasn't owned a bikini since she was a little girl, and who comes to me for a breast augmentation so she can wear one (she brings with her the three she's considering) on her upcoming trip to Mexico with her new boyfriend. Will they live happily ever after? Who knows? Will she feel sexier around him? You bet. However deep-seated our basic natures are, I can say, from years of doing this, that when body anxiety is removed by fixing the exterior, it's as if a new person—a person with a new *interior*—can finally emerge. And focus on other things, things beyond the body.

Here's the irony: So many of the patients I see come to me not because they're vain—the common perception—but because they *don't want* to be thinking about their body and face! They want to be consumed by the world outside, not the world that begins and ends with their skin.

That's why I became a surgeon. To watch people become more alive. To make them happier.

Everything I've said in the last page or so is as true, potentially, of someone who feels wrinkled, old, and unattractive as it is of someone whose face has been mangled by a car accident. Our goal as plastic surgeons is to make people happy. Period. So if I can make a woman whose husband walked out on her look terrific and feel confident about her appearance . . . she's probably experiencing at least as big a jolt in her life as someone who had me revise a scar from a childhood operation.

▼

The vice president at Blythedale Children's Hospital in Westchester—the mother of a patient of mine—approached me about starting a reconstructive program for children with severe deformities and malformations. I was immediately excited by the idea. Over the next week, I started to jot down notes about requirements for the program. I was unsure about how the endeavor would be funded until one night when I was seated at a New York restaurant, eagerly describing to my date the possibilities for the program. A diner seated behind me overheard our conversation. She leaned over, introduced herself as Ann Colley, and said, "I apologize for interrupting, but I think I know someone who can help you out."

Ann Colley is an angel.

The next day, a woman introducing herself only as Janet telephoned my office. "I work for a gentleman who is very successful on Wall Street," said Janet. "He's a religious and thankful man. He has four healthy children, and he wants to give something back to society. But he only wants to donate to charities where the money goes completely to the children. And he wants it to be anonymous."

Janet, as his representative, came to inspect the hospital. Within ten minutes, she asked to leave, with tears in her eyes. Blythedale is a unique place that makes you realize just how lucky you are to have your health.

An hour after reaching her office, Janet called back, pledging millions of dollars on behalf of the mystery benefactor.

"My boss was so impressed," she said, "I'm sure that his friends would also like to help to fund this endeavor."

There were never forms to fill out. Just a single telephone call.

There really is a God.

To date, we have been frugal with the money, and these generous benefactors have helped many people regain the use of their arms, their legs, their lives. We've worked on many children who have suffered terribly disfiguring conditions, but a couple of them stand out. Ronnie Lugo, who didn't have a home and was living on the street, was thirteen years old when he had acid thrown in his face. It horribly scarred him, restricted his jaw movement, and cost him sight in his left eye. I reconstructed his eyelid with a series of flaps and skin grafts. The *New York Times* became interested in Blythedale and ran a story describing our program. An ophthalmologist at Columbia University read the story and called me up.

"Dr. Lesesne?" he said. "I read about your boy in the *New York Times*. I have a new procedure that I think can restore his eyesight."

Ronnie had his surgery a month later and went from wanting to kill himself to wanting to be a child psychologist.

Another case was at once satisfying and hugely disappointing—but the disappointment had nothing to do with the limits of medicine or surgery. Kevin, a two-year-old boy, had suffered burns on 40 percent of his body. He was so scarred, he wasn't growing and he couldn't walk. He could not stretch out his knees because of his flexion/contraction scars. I did multiple skin grafts, scar releases, and Z-plasties—a technique that reverses the direction of a scar to allow skin around it to grow again. Kevin started to walk again. He started to grow again. He started to play baseball again.

A couple of years later, another boy was brought into our clinic who had been similarly profoundly burned. Naturally, the boy and his family were distraught, and I thought it would help their psyches tremendously if the family of Kevin, who was doing spectacularly well now, would talk to these people and offer words of encouragement and show them there were reasons for hope. I called Kevin's father and told him what I needed.

"No," he said.

"No?" I said.

"That part of Kevin's life is over. We want nothing to do with burn victims or anything that reminds us of burn victims. That part of our life is over."

The second boy, fortunately, also had a relatively successful surgical outcome.

But while I understand that some people want to put the past behind them, I will never forgive Kevin's father for not talking to another family going through the distress that his family had, when they had been fortunate enough to make it to the other side of their despair. To this day, when I think about that phone call, I can almost feel my blood boil.

Even though the vast majority of my practice was in-office cosmetic surgery, every so often I would find myself doing a surgery that was almost surreal.

Edward came to see me at his sister's recommendation (she'd had a rhinoplasty years before). He had a small lump on his left eyebrow that he wanted me to examine and possibly remove. The moment I dissected around it, I was concerned. The lump had a gray, gritty consistency. From its appearance, a sarcoma was highly probable.

The biopsy results came back positive for cancer—specifically, "spindle-cell" sarcoma, something very rare that I'd only heard of, never seen. I had to research it on Medline, an online search engine for doctors. The cancer grows along the sheath of the nerve. It's highly malignant.

I discussed the situation with Edward, gently telling him the bad news, the treatment, the future. I told him that this could be bad, lethal. He was amazingly calm about it; his family was not. A CT scan revealed that the cancer had tunneled above his eye and traveled to the roof of the orbit, the bony wall around the eye. I suggested we remove the cancer immediately.

After a tedious dissection of Edward's face, I kept finding more cancer.

And more.

And more.

And more.

It was as if the cancer were flowing along a stream; the stream was the nerve. I couldn't tell just by looking whether the samples I was sending to the pathology lab were cancerous, but the results kept coming back with the unhappy verdict of "positive margins," meaning the cancer was still there, in every tissue sample I'd cut away so far.

I dissected farther to the back of the orbit and kept finding more cancer. Over three hours, I removed at least sixteen tissue samples. The cancer tracked over the eye, back deeper and deeper into his head.

The eye needed to be removed.

Since I'd never before taken out an eyeball, I called in an ophthalmologist to do the "enucleation"—permanent removal of the eye.

For all that I had prepared Edward—and myself—neither of us had had any idea, preoperatively, that we would be dealing with something this extensive, something that had already cost him one eye.

But the cancer wasn't finished. The diseased nerve tunneled down to the side of the orbit; I had to saw through cheekbone to trace the meandering nerve. It was still coming up "positive margins." I removed pieces of cheekbone but the nerve was heading back to the brain. I could not get a clear margin.

After removing much of Edward's left cheek (the incision went from the middle of his lip to the base of his nose, around the base, then through the junction of nose and cheek, and underneath his lower eyelid, so I could peel back the skin, muscles, and blood vessels), I removed the whole cheekbone, only to see that the cancerous nerve continued toward the brain, ending at its base.

Finally, after yet another tissue sample was sent in, I got back a report of "clear margins."

Now I had to close him—but how? The left side of his face had a huge hole in it. The flap options—latissimus, trapezius, deltoid—all had disadvantages. I decided to harvest a flap of tissue from his trapezius.

The surgery took thirteen hours.

For two weeks, Edward lay in the ICU. Finally, he was well enough to leave the hospital. He consulted an oncologist.

He was—all things considered—improving. He resumed a near normal life.

Many months later, he started getting pain in his left scalp. A CT scan revealed that the cancer had returned. It had probably infiltrated to his brain.

He came to see me, asking for my recommendation.

"I don't know if anyone can get around it," I said. I advised against having another operation.

Edward found a surgeon in Los Angeles who took off the front half of Edward's skull. In the OR, Edward suffered cardiac arrest. He remained in the ICU for six months. He died.

During his remaining months, he could have lived without the surgery. No matter what, he would have been in pain at the end. Yet that would almost certainly have been a better fate than the one he suffered, and better for his family, too.

When a surgeon advises you not to operate, consider it seriously.

You Want What?

▼ ▼ ▼

Dennis, a computer hardware salesman in his early thirties, came in for a consult. He said he wanted to change his looks.

"Okay," I said. "What do you want?"

"Actually, I want a lot."

"Like what?"

"I want to look like Jennifer Aniston."

It didn't register. Jennifer Aniston? Who's that?

"She's an actress," he said. "Don't you watch TV? She's my absolute favorite of all time."

"Apparently. When you say you want to look like her . . . how much?"

"*Exactly* like her," said Dennis. He told me that for almost a year he'd been taking estrogen. He wanted me to do several procedures—cheek, chin, and breast implants. And the big, nonreversible penectomy.

Much as I was sympathetic and wanted to help Dennis, I declined his request. I could have done the smaller procedures, but I'd never done a penectomy, which involves removal of the penis, then rotation of the excess skin of the penis to create a vagina. I'd assisted in constructing vaginas while I was a resident at Stanford—a technically difficult procedure that presents such challenges as infection and scar tissue buildup in a sensitive area.

I referred Dennis to a clinic seasoned at gender-swapping surgeries and wished him well.

Everybody's got something that bothers him or her.

▼

It's hard sometimes not to say outright to a patient, "No, you're wrong. I'm right. Trust me on this and *don't have this surgery.*" I don't say that as much as I should because it sounds arrogant and the patient probably wouldn't listen anyway. Martina, a postsurgical transsexual who'd had multiple operations (over five years, I'd done her nose, eyes, face, neck, breasts, and legs), returned to ask me to remove two lower ribs. I wouldn't. The surgery would leave a prominent scar. Deeper structures, such as the liver, could be injured. The improvement in shapeliness was not worth the risk. Since Martina and I had a history, and since there's always another plastic surgeon out there who *will* do surgery no matter how ill-advised, I tried to persuade her to reconsider.

"You'll hate the scar," I predicted. "It's not worth it."

My oratorical skills were apparently less treasured than my surgical ones, and Martina had someone else remove the ribs.

She liked the new contour all right. She hated the scar.

Obviously I'm a proponent of plastic surgery. But a successful surgery is not a given, no matter how good the doctor or how simple the procedure. There's a continuum of human psychology, and those who exist at one end of the continuum won't ever set foot in my office, while those at the other end I'm well-advised to rebuff. That is, if a patient doesn't care, or is in denial, about her appearance, she'll never consider plastic surgery. And if a patient is self-absorbed or narcissistic, she'll never deem the surgery a success.

The best candidates for plastic surgery fall somewhere within these extremes, with a healthy enough mix of self-esteem and humility to make the chances for a successful surgery plausible.

▼

A couple years after his initial visit, I got a call from Dennis, the man who'd wanted me to help make him look like Jennifer Aniston. He wanted to see me about some work.

When he appeared in my office, his look was considerably softer and he was (in his words) "more than halfway" toward looking like his favorite actress. He was post–psychological evaluation and still taking hormones, and he wanted me to perform four operations: breast implants, cheek implants, rhinoplasty, and eyelift. I was much more comfortable working on him now.

He was happy with the results. Afterward, he said he was off, finally, to have his dream transgender operation. I wished him well again, and again he disappeared.

It's a huge compliment when someone entrusts you to make him or her look better. It's an even greater compliment when they trust you to lead them to a new life—a new profession, a new way of living. Michael, a nice-looking forty-year-old electronics specialist for General Motors, wanted to be Elvis. "Before you tell me I'm crazy and order me to leave your office," he said, though I'd made no move to do so, nor had I thought to, "I'm *not* crazy. If the surgery puts *anything* in jeopardy, I won't do it. I'm happily married, I have two great kids, I love my family, I have a good job. But it's my dream in life to be an Elvis impersonator. I can do everything Elvis can—sing, dance, I sound like him. You won't believe how much I sound like him. But I don't look like him. To get an act in Vegas or Atlantic City, I need to look like him."

He seemed thoughtful, not a kook. Before or since, I have not encountered a more levelheaded, self-aware, inspiring justification for elective cosmetic surgery.

To make a patient look like someone else requires a different mind-set. I get about four such requests a year—sometimes to look like a celebrity (Sharon Stone's a favorite), sometimes to get a favorite celebrity feature (Andie MacDowell's eyes, Angelina Jolie's lips), sometimes to look like some attractive stranger whose photo the patient has brought along. As a surgeon, I have to take an unusual approach. First, I have to forget my own aesthetics, since the point is not to make the patient look better but to look different. Second, I have to be sure the look we're going for is feasible given the patient's facial structure. Third, I need to figure out just how close I can get to the patient's ideal.

That night, while making sketches and planning what Michael would require to look like Elvis, it struck me that we first had to make a choice. Elvis . . . but at what age? Young Elvis or old Elvis? The twentyish hearththrob Elvis? The thirtyish, more mature Elvis? The fortyish, paunchier, Vegas Elvis? The post office had ultimately issued two stamps, from different eras. We had no such luxury.

Not surprisingly, Michael had already given it lots of thought. In his late thirties, he knew his options were limited. Together, he and I looked through Elvis album covers. We found the perfect blueprint on one of his gospel albums, when Elvis was in his mid- to late thirties. I made a copy of the cover and placed a grid on it. Then I photographed Michael's face, enlarged the photo to match the album, put the same grid on it, and superimposed it on the album. I measured centimeters, millimeters. I noted how to change his nose, eyes, cheeks, lips, and chin.

Six operations later, including two for the cheeks, Michael and I, between us, had re-created Elvis. Yet one thing kept gnawing at me: Despite Michael's uncanny resemblance to the King, despite all the planning, despite two follow-ups, I never quite got the left dimple the way I wanted it.

On Michael's final post-op visit before he and his supportive family were to move to Las Vegas, as he sat in my waiting room wearing shades, slicked hair, sideburns, and GM work clothes, a woman accompanied by her two children entered. When the girl saw Michael, her mouth hit the floor.

"*Mommy!*" she whispered, loud as a yell. "*It's Elvis!*"

The mother did an impressive double take. Now the little boy stared, too. Michael, overflowing with delight, turned his back on them for a moment, rolled his hips, then peeked back at them over his shoulder and pointed at the girl. "*Helloooo,* little girl," he said in a lowered voice.

The King lives. Michael legally changed his last name to Vegas and he now performs regularly in Las Vegas and Atlantic City.

It still bugs me that I didn't get the dimple.

"I want Texas tits!" announced Marilyn, a big, pretty new consult from Dallas, as if she were ordering a burger.

Marilyn, single and thirty-five, was not like the bulk of my Texas patients, who tended to go for a less "bold" look than Marilyn. Then again, Dolly Parton might go for a less bold look than Marilyn.

Texas tits, to Marilyn, meant breast implants seven hundred cubic centimeters big—large by any standard. Normally, I would have told her no, outright, or that I would do an implant but not quite so large. And it was not about my aesthetic vision being different from hers. At the volume she was contemplating, breast size may become a health issue; she might have been inviting back pain.

But Marilyn wasn't a small girl at all. Seven hundred cubic centimeters is proportional only to a tall, broad-shouldered woman, and she could handle it. It fit her physique.

More to the point, it's what she wanted.

Still, I tried to dissuade her. But she insisted that was the look she wanted. "I know they'll work," she said.

"It's going to be a 38D, at least," I replied.

"I don't care. That's what I want."

I've never augmented a woman that large, before or since.

A year later, while walking down Park Avenue, I noticed a tall, attractive woman approaching. She was nicely dressed and pushing a baby carriage. As she neared, she looked more familiar, but it didn't quite click for me. As she came closer, I finally recognized her, and she me. She broke into a big smile. We stopped.

"It worked," she said. "He's two months old. That was the best investment I ever made."

I smiled at her, and then at the baby.

"Dr. Lesesne?" she said.

"Yes?"

"I wonder what else I can do."

I looked at her, confused.

"I'm sure," she said, "that there are other procedures I need."

I smiled at her. I didn't know what to say.

Soon, she walked away, pushing the baby carriage up Park Avenue.

In my mail was an envelope from California, with no return address. I opened it and unfolded the single sheet inside. It was a copy of a California driver's license. The license photo was of a woman who looked very much like Jennifer Aniston, only more angular, longer in the face.

The first name on the license? Jennifer.

Dennis, you did it.

I Don't Do That

▼ ▼ ▼

In the late nineties, referrals between East Coast and West Coast became more frequent, and the entertainment portion of my clientele increased. I was visited by Susan, wife of one of America's most beloved entertainers (he started as a singer, then eventually won recognition for his acting and comic talents). I had done a face-lift on Susan's friend that Susan had admired, and now she had come in from California for the same procedure.

She came to my office by herself. No putting on airs, I was pleased to note, though Susan certainly had the money and last name to go that route.

We talked briefly, and I told her how much I'd loved her husband's work when I was growing up and how much I still loved it. Then I looked at her and we started to talk about what I would do, and she listened intently.

"Now I'll need to get a couple of old photos of you so I can examine and study how you've aged," I concluded.

"No, you won't," she said.

"Yes, I need a few photos of earlier and now. For the new photos, you can keep the negatives and send me the prints. It helps me to get the most natural look."

"Absolutely not."

"I need photos to study. To do the job right."

"You can do it without photographs."

"No, actually, I can't. You look different lying down. Gravity pulls skin in a different fashion. I might not be able to see what's truly fatty or not. That's why I need to analyze photos."

"There will be no photos," she said.

Life is too short for certain things. And in this case, the risks of a mistake and an unsatisfied patient were great.

"I don't think this is going to work out," I told her, polite as could be.

She stood, turned, and walked out, mumbling under her breath, "What does *he* know?"

Surgeons love to do surgery. It's worth seriously considering that fact when a surgeon says that he or she won't operate.

There are various reasons to turn prospective patients down.

Physical: There's just not enough there that needs fixing. (In short: If I can't see it, I can't fix it.)

Psychological: I sense that the patient is incapable of being made happy by *any* surgery, no matter how well executed. Or, as in the case of Susan, there's a lack of rapport and trust between the patient and me.

Comfort level: I now only do procedures I've done hundreds or thousands of times.

Interest level: I don't do procedures that don't interest me. For example, I simply have no desire to do hair transplants. I don't do hymen repairs—elevating a flap of the vagina lining and suturing it across the opening to the other side—though I've had numerous calls from Arabic men (from Kuwait City, Cairo, and Lebanon) asking me to do a reconstruction for a sister or female friend. In Arabic countries (among other places), they believe that having such a procedure will make the woman more desirable for marriage, as it purports to attest to her virginity.

Nor am I interested in vaginal tightening—cutting out tissue to reduce the diameter of the vaginal opening.

I also won't do procedures that have a high dissatisfaction rate.

For me, these include pectoral implants, buttock implants, and circumferential body lifts. This last operation—where you cut all around the stomach and lift the legs—requires working on an extremely large surface area, there's a lot of bleeding, and the scar is disfiguring. A colleague of mine, a good surgeon, recently did a circumferential body lift and had complications. I thought, *If it can happen to him, it can happen to me.* (Interestingly, though, in studying the circumferential body lift, I discovered a better way to do a thighplasty, which frees me from having to go completely around the body and involves less scarring. Yet another example of why you must constantly keep up on what's going on in the profession.)

Penile augmentation also has a high failure rate. It's difficult to put foreign material (in this case, AlloDerm) into the shaft of the penis without a high risk of scarring and infection. This is another surgery I won't do.

Joanna and Theresa brought in their eight-year-old daughter, Amy, whose ears were large and sticking out. Correcting the ears would not be hard; dealing with the two mothers (Theresa was the birth mom) would be.

"There must be a way you can use a holistic anesthesiologist," Joanna kept insisting. I said, again, that for many years I'd operated side by side with one of a couple of trusted anesthesiologists, and that I much preferred to work with them.

"There's a CD that Amy would like you to play when you're operating," Theresa said more than once, even though I'd told them I don't like music or distractions in my OR.

The questions and issues kept coming. This was our fourth consultation. Poor Amy looked so nervous that I thought, if I were to do the procedure, we'd probably sedate her rather than use the local we normally give. The women asked more questions than I'd been asked by any single patient in twenty years of practice.

I didn't have the stomach for a fifth consultation.

"I'm sorry, but I don't think I'm your surgeon," I said. "I don't feel comfortable doing the surgery."

"But we want you," Joanna said.

"Yes, we want you," Theresa said.

I held my ground.

The next day I got a call from the father—at least, the sperm donor—of the girl.

"They really want you," he said.

I told him it was best that I passed.

America's Sweetheart
▼ ▼ ▼

In the summer of 1999, Janice, an agent for TV personalities, came to see me about a growth on her face. After I removed it for a biopsy (it would turn out to be benign), she asked me if I was single. I was.

"I have someone you should meet," she said. "Katie Couric."

I nodded. "Who's Katie Couric?"

She smiled—waiting, I later realized, for me to smile at my obvious put-on.

"You don't know who Katie Couric is?" she said.

"No."

"You're joking, right?"

"I'm not," I said. "Who is she?"

Janice stared at me sideways, as if making extra sure I wasn't pulling her leg. When I say I don't get out much, I mean it.

"That's so perfect," she said, accepting my word finally. "She's a TV news anchor."

"I don't watch TV," I said.

Janice shook her head and chuckled. "That's so perfect."

I scribbled Ms. Couric's phone number on my prescription pad. A week later, with great hesitation, I called her at home. I know blind dates can work (though the odds are not good), but I wasn't used to that kind of near anonymous setup and didn't want to make a fool of myself.

I shrugged it off. How much harm was there in getting together for a cup of coffee with the TV person? On the phone, I awkwardly introduced myself. With each sentence, though, I felt more comfortable, and a marvelous thing happened: What I'd expected to be a brief chat to set time and place for coffee turned into a two-hour conversation. We had mutual friends from the University of Virginia, where Katie had gone to college, and also in the media world. After twenty minutes I realized I was talking with the world's most wonderful, easygoing conversationalist—which would not have surprised morning-TV-watching America, given what Katie has done so well for so many years. To me, though, it was a revelation. I wasn't infatuated but was certainly curious.

A few evenings later, I sat at a little bistro off Madison Avenue, getting stood up. Six thirty, our appointed time, came and went, then 6:45 and 7:00. At 7:15, tired of wasting my time and a little miffed, I finally left. Not three paces into my walk uptown, a black limousine pulled alongside me. The window rolled down. It was Katie. Nice timing. She apologized profusely for being late.

"Are you hungry?" she asked, and I said I was. "Forget coffee," she said. "Let's go to my favorite restaurant."

She got out and we walked to Coco Pazzo, on Seventy-fourth and Madison. As soon as we entered, everyone, it seemed, came over to greet her. She was New York royalty. I'd been out with notable women before, but never someone this recognizable. We were given a quiet table for two. Katie didn't bother to look at the menu. "What are you having?" I asked.

"Nothing," she said. "I've eaten dinner with my children."

Over (my) dinner, she told me, for the next hour and a half, about her kids, whom she obviously adored, and about her late husband, Jay, and his battle with colon cancer, which had ended a year and a half before. (After his death, Katie used the *Today* show to raise national awareness about colon cancer, even televising her own colonoscopy.) I liked listening to her talk. I couldn't help but smile at the role reversal: As she told her stories and shared her thoughts, I was experiencing the exact opposite of what Katie Couric does all the time, when she asks the questions and listens to the responses. It was clear that she had not yet healed from the loss of her husband, and I think that my ability—any good physician's ability—to provide a sympathetic ear was a balm to her.

By the end of our hour-and-a-half meal, I had long ago forgotten her tardiness.

After dinner, we walked down Madison Avenue for a block until I stuck out my hand to say good night. "Let's walk a few blocks," she said. We could not advance more than fifty feet without a fan recognizing her, or an acquaintance coming up to say hello. Each time they did, I retreated several steps. She was clearly comfortable with her fame, but I did not want to intrude on it. After walking six blocks, I again stuck out my hand to say good night. "I really should go," I said.

"Let's walk a little more," she said.

I guess things were going well, though I wasn't sure. I walked her to her building and stuck my hand out once more.

"Aren't you at least going to walk me up to my door? What's wrong with you Princeton men? Even we Virginians know better than that."

Red-faced, I walked her upstairs and gave her a peck on the cheek.

I wasn't sure what to make of the date. The next day I called Janice to thank her for introducing us and told her I liked Katie. "Well, I think she likes you," Janice said. Given all my supposed insight into the opposite sex, I should have understood that "I think she likes you" means "She likes you." Instead, I just thought that, you know, she liked me.

I called for a second date, this time dinner for *both* of us. After a day of performing surgery, I walked over to her place. She had just come from spending the afternoon with her kids. She and I walked into the early twilight of a New York summer evening, one of those magical times where the city almost feels as if it's flaunting how romantic it can be.

"Let's walk up the avenue and see which restaurants look good," I said.

As we strolled, Katie and I talked, in a jokey way, about how this could really work out between us. She had to be up for work at five; so did I. She didn't really drink; neither did I. Professionally, we seemed equally driven. The conversation was, as it apparently couldn't *but* be with her, delightful and fast-paced and constant. One indication to me that I liked her was that my PSR was turned off. My first impression of her, physically, was that she was extremely cute but a little shorter than my type. And like any plastic surgeon—like any man—I started to scan her face for the quick readout. But none came. No "bone structure this" or "jawline that." My radar simply stayed off. And that's not meant to be a backhanded compliment.

We passed a charming French restaurant on Eighty-ninth Street but decided it was too beautiful an evening to be inside; it was a night made for sipping wine in Central Park. I poked my head inside the restaurant and told the maître d' what I wanted—and he told me, with regrets, that it's against the law in New York City for a restaurant to sell a bottle of wine to take out. I tried to coerce him but he wouldn't budge. I pulled out the one trump card that always works with the French: French. I pleaded with him in his language. *C'est notre deuxième rendez-vous, monsieur,* I told him. (This is our second date.) *Regardez, comment elle est jolie!* (Look how pretty she is!) *N'est-elle pas adorable?* (Isn't she adorable?) Katie had no idea what I was saying or at least she smiled graciously and played dumb, but the maître d' finally cracked. Feeling sorry for me—and appreciating the Gallic lengths to which I was going for romance—he sold me a bottle of his best cabernet and two glasses to go, and

Katie and I headed for the park. We never reached it. We commandeered a bench on Sixty-eighth Street, just outside the park, opened our bottle, and drank wine and talked for hours as the world passed by. This time, no one approached Katie. I don't know if it was dumb luck, or if everyone was in his own world on this gorgeous night, or if she and I were just in our own cocoon. But it was simplicity itself. At the end of the evening, I walked her all the way back to her place—ever the good Princeton man this time—and kissed her on the cheek.

I was warming to her. It had been an inarguably great beginning to what might become a wonderful relationship.

While I found my romantic life improving, professionally I found myself facing one of the greatest challenges of my career, a somewhat ironic one at the moment: I was determined to help one of my patients to get just one date.

Natalie, fifteen years old, was wheelchair-bound from growth abnormalities in her spine. She also suffered from agenesis of the mandible—meaning she'd been born without a lower jaw. The condition caused her to drool and her speech to be garbled. Before I saw her, she had undergone several operations to reconstruct the jaw with "nonvascularized" bone grafts. This means that blood vessels were not directly attached to the new bone. Without the blood vessels, these grafts reabsorbed over time. Scar tissue developed in the area and she would require a more major, cutting-edge procedure and treatment. The plan was to harvest a free fibular graft from her leg and attach it to the blood vessels (an artery and two veins) in her neck. This would create a lower jaw with its own blood supply. With the better blood flow, the bone would survive, grow, and one day allow artificial teeth to be implanted. Natalie couldn't really smile, but her eyes could. She was excited about the operation. Her new jaw would not only give her a prettier face, but would allow her to eat more normally. For Natalie, though, that was secondary. Like any teenager, she wanted to go out on a date. She wanted to go on a date more than anything else in the world. I promised her that if she didn't get a date in six months, I'd help her find one. Her eyes lit up. I told her we were embarking together on this journey to reconstruct her jaw.

The operation involved certain techniques I no longer did frequently. I recommended her to a team at New York University that specialized in bone-graft microsurgery. They performed the operation, after which Natalie was sent back to the children's hospital in Westchester, where she could heal and rehabilitate.

At least, that was the idea.

In the late summer and early fall, Katie and I went on several more dates, usually in quiet restaurants, sitting away from the crowd. She seemed happy to take things slow, keep it low-key. I respected the special and delicate position her celebrity often put her in. We spoke on the phone nearly every day.

One afternoon, she suggested we go that night to Elaine's, the renowned Upper East Side establishment. I agreed, but wondered aloud at the wisdom of frequenting such a public place. To top it off, that evening, before I met Katie, I had the gathering sense that I was being followed. By whom, I couldn't tell. But twice I saw a gray car gliding slowly down the street, a proper distance behind me. (New York cars not in traffic never move that slowly unless they're trolling for a parking space.) At first, I suspected it might be someone associated with the politician from Istanbul on whom I'd just done a necklift. She was spending the night, postoperatively, at the Waldorf. Giselle, one of my two private-duty nurses, was going to spend the night in the hotel suite caring for her. As Giselle and I took a cab down to the Waldorf, I shared my suspicion that we were being tailed.

"You're paranoid," she told me.

After stopping in at the suite to check on my patient, I left Giselle to meet Katie at her building—and now I was more convinced than ever that I was being followed, this time on foot. Leaving the Waldorf, I walked over to Lexington Avenue. At one point, I turned, and a man about thirty yards behind me stopped, looked momentarily fitful, then disappeared randomly into the nearest store.

But why would he be working for my Turkish patient, tucked away in her hotel room and healing nicely? What was the point in tailing me *after* the operation? Maybe it was an agent for another powerful patient-to-be, making sure I was professional and discreet, not a drinker and a weirdo? Before their employer committed to come see me? It wouldn't be the first time. I had clients whose security people had me ship them my Botox and collagen, in an Igloo container, in a 727 provided by them, so that their own chemists could make sure I wasn't going to poison their majesties.

I caught a taxi back downtown, still haunted by the feeling that someone was watching—so much so that I had the cabdriver drop me off blocks from Katie's building. I walked this way and that to make sure I had rid myself of any followers, not quite serpentining.

At Katie's building, I again asked her about the wisdom of going to Elaine's. "Are you sure you want this?" I said. "Once we set foot in there, word gets around."

"I don't care," she said.

At Elaine's, we met friends of Katie's and had a wonderful evening.

Walking back to her place afterward, Katie said, "Aren't you going to put your arm around me?"

This time I did so without hesitation. It was funny to me that she was much more comfortable with our being publicly affectionate than I was. After dropping her off at her place, I was about to exit the lobby . . . when something told me not to. Instead, I went out the side entrance.

A few days later, Katie called me. A security guy at NBC News, she said, had received an anonymous call saying, "Cap Lesesne is trouble. Katie Couric should watch out."

"What's going on?" she asked me.

I told her I had no idea.

"You don't know anything about this?" she said.

"Not a clue," I said, flummoxed and disturbed. "I have no idea."

She was completely understanding. "Maybe we need to be a little more careful when we go out," she said. I agreed; that had been my stance from the beginning.

A few days later, after nine hours of surgery up in my Westchester office, I walked exhaustedly down the hall toward the exit, eager for dinner and a night's sleep. As I stepped outside, an explosion of flashbulbs went off, blinding me.

Dazed, I looked around. Five photographers stood in a small circle in the parking lot in front of me. "Hey, Doc, look here!" one of them yelled, and reflexively I did. More flashbulbs exploded. Before I could think to say anything, they were in their cars and speeding away.

Raising Eyebrows
▼ ▼ ▼

I t's impossible to say how a person will act right before an operation. You can make an educated guess, based on how they've behaved to that point—Were they insecure during the consultation? How often did they call the office in the days leading up to the surgery? How many times did they ask the same question? etc.—but even there you can just as well be dead wrong. Women tend to ask more questions than men, and waffle about what they want done—but that's *before* they've decided to go through with it. That's not what I'm talking about. I'm talking about the two crucible surgical moments: the one right before the patient is put under, and the one, post-op, when there's actual physical discomfort and pain to deal with. It's in those two moments that you find out a lot about people.

Few patients had hounded me more before an operation than Gerald, a fifty-four-year-old investment banker who had come in to discuss a browlift and an eye lift. They are two of the simpler procedures I do, and nothing about Gerald's situation made them anything other than ordinary (he had a full head of hair). But he called my staff at least twice and often three times a day, every day, for the week leading up to the surgery, and at least half those times insisted on being put through to me. He asked questions (fine, of course), then different questions (fine), then repeats of the earlier questions (still fine), then repeats of the earlier questions again (not so fine), then repeats of repeats of the later questions (enough). I was certain that right before the surgery, and then in the hours and days following, Gerald would be a pain in the ass.

But the morning of the operation, he was quiet—not frightened or morbid, just cool, ready, and confident.

I don't buy it, I thought. Then I thought, *Ha! He's saving all the complaining for afterwards!*

When the surgery was over, Gerald remained in the recovery room for ninety minutes, a standard post-op period for his procedures. No complaints, nothing. Giselle told him he could get dressed.

As he walked out the door with his daughter, he waved at me.

"We'll hear from him in about sixty seconds," I predicted to Tanya and Giselle, looking at my watch.

I heard from him once more. Three weeks later. To thank me. That was it.

Gerald was the lesson I needed just then. To remind me that life is full of surprises.

A week later, a photograph of me—tired, my hair a mess from wearing a surgeon's hat all day—appeared in all the tabloids. The *Globe,* the *Enquirer,* the *Star,* and the *New York Post* all referred to me as "Katie Couric's boyfriend," her first since the death of her husband. Rush Limbaugh noted the liaison on his radio show. Friends and patients called to chide me for looking so awful in the photograph. "Wow," one of them said. "Katie's really scraping the barrel."

I called Katie with a chagrined apology. "I'm sorry you're going out with such an unkempt dork."

"Don't worry about it," she said, but her voice was laced with more than a little concern.

"Is something wrong?" I asked.

"There may be other things to worry about."

"Like what?" I asked dumbly.

Katie told me she'd been informed by a source that my ex-wife, along with her previous ex-husband (#2), had spoken to the *Globe* about me. They were going to report that she said I had abused her.

"*What?*" I said, incredulous.

Katie wanted my side of the story.

"It's shameful," I said. "What my ex-wife and, or, her ex-husband have done is shameful."

I explained to Katie how, three years before, when things were particularly sour between Elsie and me, we'd gotten into a fierce argument. (In retrospect, we'd argued too frequently for our marriage ever to have had a chance.) I described to Katie how Elsie had thrown a liquor bottle at me. How I'd thrown her out of the house—actually, grabbed her and forcefully led her out—not just to save myself from getting conked in the head but to defuse the situation and keep her from trouble. How *I'd* been the one to call the police. But that because I had physically removed her the way I did, I was guilty of third-degree assault, a misdemeanor, and I'd spent a night in jail. How the charges had been dropped by the DA *and* my ex-wife.

End of story, I told Katie.

I'd been divorced for two years, separated for a year before that, but my ex-wife, along with another of her ex-husbands, had sniffed out that I was dating America's Sweetheart and must have been out for revenge. Or maybe just cash.

I did not know how to proceed, nor did Katie. Mostly, I was stunned. We made a halfhearted promise to talk later.

At four thirty that afternoon the phone in my office rang. "Dr. Lesesne?" a man asked.

"Yes?" I said.

"I'm from the *Globe,* and we're going to run a story that you were abusive to your ex-wife, and if we don't have a response from you by eleven tomorrow morning, we're running the story as is."

My first instinct—anyone's—was to tell him to go screw himself. But I kept calm. I got off the phone and called my lawyer to tell him what had happened. Given the facts—that I *had* been arrested, despite all the extenuating circumstances—my attorney said there was little I could do about it.

"Little?" I asked. "Or nothing?"

"Nothing," he conceded. They could pretty much spin it all they wanted, he said.

They did.

KATIE'S BOYFRIEND'S DARK SECRET PAST! shrieked the *Globe* headline. On the front page.

The story was cleverly worded to keep them just this side of libel, while sounding as provocative as could be, and doing maximum damage to me.

The following day I talked with Katie. I again explained the situation, in fine detail, and she was understanding. But she was also concerned. She had children. She was alone, still vulnerable from the loss of her husband. She was in the middle of contract negotiations with NBC.

I was more concerned. My reputation and livelihood were on the line.

By the next day, my office started getting the calls.

Cancellation. Postponement.

Reschedulings.

In the proverbial blink of an eye, my greatest love and passion—my surgical career, which I'd worked hundred-plus-hour weeks for two decades to build—was officially in free fall.

A first-time consultation—a lawyer and marathon runner named Sylvie—had miraculously *not* canceled her appointment to see me, and I was quietly grateful. I wondered if the *Globe* story had escaped her notice, or if she had seen it and didn't care. I wasn't about to quiz her. She had a mild case of saddlebags that she wanted removed, fast.

Sure, I can do that, Sylvie, totally routine, we just lipo the fat from your outer legs, you'll look great . . . but first a question: Have you not been inside a supermarket the past twenty-four hours?

"When would you like to schedule that?" I asked, choosing not to point out, either, that my operating schedule in the upcoming days and weeks had suddenly become quite free.

Are you okay having me operate on you, Sylvie, what with the tabloid press and all? Or do you believe they've taken liberties with the truth?

"Well, I . . . ," she said, and now she looked down at her hands. I could see she was blushing.

Oh no. Here it comes. Brace yourself, Lesesne.

"I just started dating someone . . . ," Sylvie said, trying again. She looked me straight in the eye.

"Okay," I said.

"Well, once you do the operation," said Sylvie, ". . . how long will it be before he can put his hands on me?"

I wanted to hug her.

"Three days," I told her, and we scheduled her for that Tuesday, so they'd have the weekend.

Two days after the *Globe* story appeared, my office phone rang. This time, it was the *New York Post*—and they weren't calling to sell me a subscription.

"On Friday we're going to run a story about you and the abuse charge," they told me. The same garbage the *Globe* ran, nothing new. "And," they told me, "we're going to put you on the front page."

Again, I desperately wanted to yell "Bastard!" But I held my tongue. Again I called my lawyer, to let him deal with it. Again, he said there wasn't much to be done.

After I hung up with him, I walked out to my waiting room, shaken. It was empty. Tanya, my office manager, was wrapping up a phone call with yet another patient who wanted to reschedule.

Tanya looked up at me, her eyes glistening with tears. "Dr. Lesesne, will we have a job next week?"

I was in something approaching shock. "We'll get through this," I said, summoning my training as a doctor to stay calm, be rational, not panic. "Worse things have happened, Tanya. Whatever *does* happen, I guarantee your salary, Deanna's, and Giselle's for the next six months. We'll get through it."

It sounded nice, and I thought I believed what I said . . . but it wasn't going to stop Friday from coming. The *Post* hit the newsstands. The front page? A picture of me under the headline KATIE's BOYFRIEND SHOCKER.

Charming. I thought of my parents back in Michigan. Of my grandmother. Not that I needed to explain anything to them; they knew the details, the backstory. But still.

My attorney informed me, with regret, that we had to let the story run its course. Just ride it out, he said.

Easy for you to say, I thought. *As soon as we hang up the phone, only one of us can continue his day below the tabloid radar.*

If they were going to cloak the incident between my ex-wife and me in sinister, leading language that always stopped short of libel, my lawyer continued, then there was nothing I could really do to fight it.

So *this* is why noncelebrities have PR agents! I considered hiring one that very afternoon, but the damage was done.

There were more cancellations. One surgery candidate called

to assure Tanya that she would most certainly be going through with her face-lift but merely wanted to "wait until Dr. Lesesne is at a more stable stage in his life."

My relationship with Katie was noticeably cooling. I was growing remote, and she hardly seemed in it for the long haul. I couldn't tell how much of the distance was the result of the bad press, how much the natural evolution of our relationship. If nothing else, at least Howard Stern was on my side: While I was driving to Westchester, I heard him wonder aloud on his radio show why I was being slammed when the charges were dismissed and all that the tabloids had to go on were my wife's misleading allegations, nothing more. He told Robin to get me on the air.

"Get that Italian Dr. Luh-*sain*-ee on here to defend himself!" he implored her.

More than ever, the operating room was my sanctuary. I'd remembered reading about how when Michael Jordan was going through especially hard times—after the murder of his father, in particular, but also just the constant, everyday demands he faced as a walking, talking legend (not that I'm comparing myself to him)—he loved playing basketball more than ever. The moment he stepped over the line and onto the court, no one could get to him. Not media, not agents, not lawyers or family or friends or hangers-on or strangers. It was just him, the players, the refs, the ball, the basket, the job to do, the confidence that he would get it done.

I understood. I had always loved doing surgery; on those rare occasions when I was sufficiently ill that I had to postpone a surgery, I was irritated less from being under the weather and far more because I was deprived of doing my favorite thing in the world. But I had never looked so forward to doing surgery as I did during my tabloid hell. In the OR it was just me, the patient, my staff, the room, the objective. It's pull was so strong that I was reminded of a breast reduction I'd assisted on in med school. Dr. Nicholas Georgiade, chief of plastic surgery at Duke, never lost his way. So when he paused for several seconds midoperation, we all noticed. Behind his mask he had turned clammy and gray. "Dr. G, are you okay?" I asked.

"Fine," he said, and continued to operate, doing his usual stellar job. When the surgery was over, he walked down the hall and checked himself into a bed. During the operation, he had suffered a massive heart attack.

Now, during these difficult months, I could still concentrate as well in the OR as when my mind had been less burdened by outside things. I concentrated even better, in fact, as focused as the point of my scalpel. I craved getting immersed in the details of the operation. The measuring, the marking, the incisions, the dissecting, the shaping, the suturing . . .

When I wasn't in the OR, I worked. I prepared lectures that for years I hadn't found time to do. I read more professional texts and medical journals than usual.

Anything but the newspapers.

It was bad news. Very bad.

For almost six weeks since her operation, Natalie—the fifteen-year-old, wheelchair-bound girl who'd been born without a lower jaw—had been rehabilitating nicely from her jaw surgery, at Blythedale Children's Hospital in Westchester, in anticipation of her new life and her first-ever date. But one day on my rounds, I noticed she had saliva coming out below her jawline, dripping down her neck. I recommended that she be transferred back to NYU, where they would have to operate again.

She was transported down to the hospital. I figured she'd be there for a while, then sent back up to Westchester for an uncomplicated recovery.

A few days later, after spending the morning in the Cornell Medical School library researching a lecture I would be giving to residents on analyzing the nose, I took a cab to NYU for a "morbidity/mortality" conference, a monthly meeting in which doctors review recent cases, complications, even deaths in the hospital.

The doctor began his presentation. "We have one service mortality. Female, fifteen, suffering from both agenesis of the mandible and . . ."

I didn't hear the rest of it. I felt short of breath. After blinking a few times, I looked across the room and saw the microsurgeon who had performed Natalie's surgery. He had tears in his eyes.

It turned out that, unknown to any of us, when I discovered Natalie had saliva below her jawline, she had developed a "fistula"—an abnormal connection—in her neck, where the incisions met. Saliva was draining, inside her, from her mouth into the left side of her neck, and the digestive enzymes in her saliva were eroding her carotid artery. It was impossible to tell that just by looking at her. She had no redness, no swelling; her skin looked normal. The urgency was not apparent. When she had arrived at the hospital in New York, they were minutes away from getting her to the OR when the nurse came to her room to find her in a pool of blood.

Her carotid had blown.

She was dead within a minute.

Natalie would never get to go on that date.

I was furious at my ex-wife, of course, her ex-husband, the *Globe,* the *New York Post,* the *Enquirer,* anything tabloid-sized . . . but besides anger I felt disappointment. I was sorry I'd brought any pain or embarrassment to my family, even though I knew I'd done nothing wrong, even though I knew they knew I'd done nothing wrong.

I suspected it would take time before the specter of the tabloid scandal would fade from the minds of some of those in my circle of clients who'd recommended me to friends. We are so entrusted—as doctors, as surgeons, as listeners—that it can seem a near miracle that people we've worked on will tell their loved ones that, yes, they, too, should put their hopes and dreams in our hands, under our scalpels.

The quality of my work needed to be unimpeachable, my manner needed to be soothing and confident and straightforward, and my standing in the community needed to be impeccable.

That last part would need some rehabilitating, no matter how blameless I was.

I was hardly the only plastic surgeon who walked, and occasionally stumbled, along this delicate line.

Through the grapevine, I heard, then subsequently read in the papers, about not one but two high-profile plastic surgeons, in other cities, who shot themselves in the same month. I heard (but didn't read) about not one but two *more* surgeons, both with practices within blocks of mine, entering psychiatric wards. In each of those four cases, I didn't know how much of a role the pressure of being an alpha surgeon had played in their downfall, but I would have been surprised to learn that it didn't play a major one, the primary one. While my tabloid debacle had had nothing to do with my work itself, I couldn't help but start to feel the stress of what I did. Usually it didn't get to me; now, it was starting to.

During the day, staff at you all the time.

At night, friends coming over in restaurants, with wide, sympathetic eyes.

I'm so sorry.

Are you okay to operate?

What a tough break, Cap. You hang in there, okay?

During the day, patients wanting you to change their appearance, to make things better.

During the night, nothing. Home, reading medical journals.

There is no room whatsoever for a mistake. Personal or professional mistakes in this field do not get hidden, at least not for long. You can never be lost.

You have a greater tendency to take your life.

I never came close to harboring the dark thoughts that some of my more troubled colleagues did. Tough as it was during this period, I told myself to do one of the things I felt I was born to do.

Put on a good face.

For all the turmoil I experienced in the weeks and months following the tabloid stories (the *Post* would honor me by putting me on their front page twice more), something very, very good came of it. Honestly. Because, cliché as it sounds, it's times like those when you get to see who your real friends are.

Mary McFadden, the dress designer, called with her sympathy and support and offered to help me in any way. My longtime friend Jeanette Longoria phoned with the same message. Diego, the Venezuelan oil magnate who had once threatened to kill me because he thought I had turned his penis black, called with uplifting words, including a standing offer to send a couple of "friends" to fly up to New York and break the necks of anyone I might deem deserving.

"I appreciate that, Diego, but it's not necessary," I said.

"Not necessary, but maybe it makes you feel better?"

"Thank you anyway, Diego."

One Saturday, Barbara Merrill, one of New York's most renowned socialites and the wife of a once-embattled investment banking legend, both of whom I'd met through my friend Jeanette, telephoned. "Cap," she said, "David and I are so sorry to read about what happened to you. As you know, several years ago David was also a victim of the press. If there's anything we can do, please let us know." I told her I'd never been so lonely. She asked me to join them for a reception at her home a few evenings later honoring Valentino, the dress designer.

As I entered Barbara and David's apartment, I was extremely nervous, nearly shaking. I was unsure how people would react to me. While I'd always been so at ease at Manhattan dinner parties, this time I was scared. But Barbara took me by the hand and walked me around the dining room to introduce me to all of her guests. Before each one she said, "This is my friend Cap Lesesne. He's a great plastic surgeon."

I'll never forget that. David came over and gave me advice like a father. No words can say how much this support meant to me, when it seemed that my "friends" were running the other way. I'd heard that the Merrills had done this kind of thing for other people, just as they'd done for me.

Good *can* triumph, as any optimist will tell you. But silver linings had been difficult to come by in the previous weeks. Fortunately, my medical training (and maybe a dollop of Sunday-school education) came through once again. The experience of having seen people die, especially children, of having seen people suffer through chronic diseases, reminded me that whatever I was going through now was, in the grand scheme of things, trivial. Just as I'd told Tanya, when I was trying to convince myself at least as much as her.

The terrible press was a body blow. The firestorm of cancellations and postponements continued. Katie and I saw each other perhaps four more times, but the mood had shifted, never to return. Just before Thanksgiving, I suggested we meet for a meal. It was awkward from the first moment. Afterward, she said she needed to get milk for her children and we walked to a supermarket on Lexington. When we got outside, she turned to me. A chill was in the air.

"I think we should cool things," she said. "You've got enough baggage to get yourself to Puerto Rico."

I paused before responding. I looked at her. She could see my brain racing to pop out a sarcastic remark. But I declined. A Princeton man is always polite.

"Maybe I'll go to the Bahamas afterward," I said.

I shook her hand and walked away.

Sounds of Music

▼ ▼ ▼

The nasty press had ceased. Since Katie and I were no longer an item, it would have been truly cruel (not to mention unusual) for the tabloids to pursue the story beyond my fifteen minutes of notoriety.

Even though my practice was starting to return, I was eager to get away, far away, even for a couple of days. I have always enjoyed professional conferences, so I decided to attend one held that year in London. Anne, a well-to-do patient, now a friend, graciously offered me the use of her London town house for my overnight.

I took a late flight, picked up a cab at Heathrow, and headed right for the house. It was in a beautiful section of the city, near the American embassy. The cabbie dropped me off in front of a lovely limestone town house near Grosvenor Square. The door was open. I could see all the way through the garden floor to the backyard.

I knocked loudly. I entered, put down my bag in the front hall, and called out hello. Hearing a voice somewhere in the back, I walked toward the back of the house, where I could see a classic English garden.

I spied a woman—maybe sixty-two, in a nearly see-through negligee—standing in the garden, in profile, with binoculars pressed to her eyes, staring intently at something, moving her head slightly back and forth, back and forth. It was not Anne, my friend and the owner of the house. I'd never seen this woman before. She was oblivious to my presence.

Realizing I'd probably seen more than was intended, I moved forward a few steps and tapped lightly on the patio door.

She still didn't turn, deeply engrossed in what she was looking at. Either that or she was deaf.

This time I tried clearing my throat.

She spoke without taking her eyes from the binoculars.

"Now you have just *got* to be Cap," she said in a husky, drawn-out Southern twang. "Anne told me y'all'd be stayin' here. Don't stand there. Whyn'tcha come on out here to the garden?"

She was so preoccupied by whatever she was looking at beyond the grounds, she seemed not to care that I saw her in her negligee (or perhaps she *wanted* me to see her in her negligee). She still had binoculars pressed to her face.

I stood there for a few seconds, not quite knowing what to do, and unable to see for myself what she was staring at.

"Cap, honey, I'm Vera," she said, and stuck out her hand while continuing to stare through the binoculars. She was from a small town in Louisiana, she said. She said she was married and then mentioned her husband's name. I recognized it as the chairman/CEO of one of the fifty largest companies in the world.

"You know why I love this house so much?" she asked from behind her binoculars.

"No," I said.

"Because it's right near the United States embassy."

"All right."

"Do you know what every United States embassy has?" Her gaze was fixed on the big, blocky building a couple hundred yards from us.

"What's that?"

"Marines. *Young* marines."

"Okay."

"And do you know what United States marines do every single morning?" she asked.

I wasn't sure I wanted to know.

"Calisthenics," she said.

She watched for several more seconds, then let down the binoculars and sighed.

Back in New York, Tanya buzzed me to say that the personal assistant of someone famous was on the line and they would not speak to her, only to me. "Who is it?" I asked.

"She won't say."

I picked up. "Dr. Lesesne speaking."

"Good morning, Doctor. I'm the personal assistant for"—she paused—"Jane Smith."

That's the best fake name they could come up with? I thought. *Either Jane Smith's assistant is new, or Jane Smith isn't all that famous.*

"Ms. Smith is interested in having plastic surgery done, as well as her male friend," the assistant said, "and she understands that you do work on people of color."

"Yes, I do. What color is Jane Smith?"

"Black. The man friend is white."

"I'd be happy to set up an appointment."

"Ms. Smith is very recognizable."

"No problem," I said. "I can stay late to see her after hours, or we can schedule something for the weekend. And her friend."

The assistant said that after hours was better, and could Ms. Smith come by at seven or eight that night? She was in town for a performance but had the evening off.

I told the assistant I'd be in my office alone, and that I'd keep the door open and the light off in the entryway, so no one could see anything. The assistant seemed pleased by that bit of cloak-and-dagger.

I was hoping Jane Smith really was high-profile—but not because I needed a celebrity fix. If she was famous, and she'd found her way to me, then it meant some people out there had stopped taking my negative press seriously. That would be one small victory to help get me out of my crabby mood.

A little after seven that night, I was doing paperwork out at Tanya's desk when the door opened and in walked . . . Jane Smith. And her male friend.

She was famous all right—one of America's most renowned and influential singers. In the flesh she looked *exactly* as she did on TV, and her gestures and manner were as bold as they were when she performed—which was highly unusual since, I have found, the private persona of public figures, especially entertainers, is often so different from the public one.

Jane Smith was definitely someone for whom there could be no effective disguise. Her hairdo, in particular, was instantly recognizable. If she did not want to be noticed, especially in New York City, then she would have to have a car shuttle her everywhere. I could see a black town car—not a limo—double-parked outside my office.

After introductions and handshakes, the three of us sat down in my office, and Jane said she wanted a little lipo.

"Are you sure?" I asked. Looking at her size 4 curves, I could see nothing to remove. "I really don't think there's anything for me to do."

In fact, she looked about twenty years younger than what I thought her real age was, and if she'd had any work done, it was astoundingly good. (Before a consultation, a patient will fill out a form that asks, among other things, for their age. Some respondents lie; many leave it blank. Because Ms. Smith had come in under a veil of secrecy, I was not going to make her fill out the form. I later found out she was fifty-eight.)

She shrugged at my response, almost relieved, possibly pleased and complimented. Her partner wanted his eyes done; that, I said, I could do. I told him I would need some photos. I would guarantee their secrecy, I assured them. I did this kind of thing all the time.

Jane smiled.

"One reason I have to be so secretive," she said, as if I actually deserved an explanation, which of course I didn't, "is I'm married. My husband lives in Florida and John here"—she took his hand—"is my friend in New York."

I told them not to worry. I opened my scheduling book, set up an appointment, gave John the relevant presurgery details, and told them how much the eyelid job would cost.

"I want to pay in cash," said Jane.

I waved my hand. "Cash, check, whatever—"

"No, no, no, not a check!" she said, and more than a flash of uneasiness crossed her eyes, as if she knew that someday, inevitably, she would slip up and get busted by her husband.

And probably the tabloids.

Two weeks later, the boyfriend came in for his eye job. Routine, went well.

Three months later, I received a handwritten note from his incredibly famous girlfriend. Two tickets were inside.

"Doctor, please come to my show at the Garden," it read. It was signed with her real name. Then it said, "P.S. Like your work. Someday, I may even need it . . . someday."

Given Jane Smith's appetite for deep cover, I assumed it was not a referral from her but rather just a coincidence that I soon got a couple more high-profile patients from the pop music world. A rock star of a metallic nature came in with his girlfriend or wife (it was unclear). She said that one of her trainers had recommended me. She wanted bigger implants than the large ones she already had.

He sported more tattoos and jewelry than anyone else who'd ever set foot in my office, probably more than any *six* people who'd ever set foot there. Behind the facade, though, he turned out to be as businesslike as a Harvard MBA. Well-spoken, focused, driven. He was a great lesson to me to not make assumptions based on what people look like.

Some luminaries in the entertainment business, you think initially, you'd love to operate on. They're younger. You know you can obtain a great result. Because of their visibility, they may help to promote your practice big-time. At first blush, the ideal patient.

Then you have your second thought, which is: Maybe this wouldn't be such a great idea, after all.

B.J. was a drummer for an extremely well-known rock group. Like any man in his late forties, B.J. did not like seeing a wattle in his neck.

"I can't believe I'm getting old like my dad," he told me. "I gotta look younger. We've got a tour coming up. What can you do?"

I told him it would be easy to liposuction his neck, though I might also have to pull the skin a bit (I'd hide the scars around the earlobes). Although his hair was shorter than it had been in his younger days, I saw no problem.

B.J. left my office having already scheduled an OR date that would leave him enough time to recover before the start of the tour.

At the end of the day, I started to make notes in his chart and review his medical history. He'd been frank. Now, it dawned on me that maybe he was a greater risk than I'd realized; a *much* greater risk. In his past, he had done more than simple recreational drugs. Because of that, he might have some underlying cardiac issues that are not always detected on routine EKGs or stress tests. Cocaine, which he'd used extensively, is notorious for causing arrhythmias.

My thought began to change from anticipated delight to anticipated dread. Instead of people thinking, *Jeez, B.J. went to Dr. Lesesne and he looks great,* now I imagined them thinking, *Jeez, B.J. went to Dr. Lesesne and had cardiac arrest and died in his office.* I could see fans of B.J. and his band stalking me.

When I left my office that night, I was not at all excited to do B.J.'s surgery. But how would I tell him? After mulling it over during the night, I thought the best tactic was to be direct.

I called him the next day. "I don't think I'm the surgeon for you. I have fears about doing your surgery that I can't shake."

Contrary to what one might think about someone with the star power of B.J., who has people constantly pampering him, he took the news intelligently. He asked appropriate questions. By the end of the phone call, he'd decided against doing the surgery altogether. He was deeply appreciative of my honesty and said he would be delighted to refer people to me (and he has).

"Maybe I'm getting old, after all," he said as we wrapped up the conversation. "But I got too many more gigs to drop dead just yet."

Soon after, a major record producer came in, a man who'd worked with virtually every big act in the music business. In his early sixties, he wasn't sitting across from me because he feared someone might take his job. He simply wanted a "tune-up"—a face-lift—because he dealt with younger people all the time.

"Nobody—let me repeat: *nobody*—can know," he told me. "Not in my business."

When he brought in photos of himself at earlier ages, practically each one showed him arm in arm with the most famous pop and rock musicians of the twentieth century.

I planned the surgery carefully with him and did a highly modified face-lift, using very short incisions. When he came in for his follow-up, he smiled. "Every now and then, Dr. Lesesne," the producer said, relaxed as could be, "you just have to give yourself a tune-up."

For an instant I forgot that he was talking about himself. I thought he was offering me advice.

He was right.

Two weeks later, I left the city bound for Tokyo, Taipei, and Hong Kong. The National Palace Museum in Taipei beckoned. Leaving New York and immersing myself in Asian art took me completely away from the turmoil back home. It was just what the doctor needed. When I returned, I threw myself into my practice even more intensely.

But the aftertaste of the whole Katie episode and the bad ending were still with me. My life seemed to have fewer people in it—fewer friends to socialize with, certainly fewer patients. I was down. I telephoned my friend Pat for dinner. She's one of those great friends who's wonderful except when you're in trouble, in which case she gets *really* wonderful.

Pat, sensing that I was low, unusual for me, invited a friend of hers named Phyllis to join us. I agreed, happy for company. The three of us dined at Demarchelier, on Eighty-sixth Street. In my distracted state, I barely noticed Phyllis, across the table.

We three talked about random things, and I felt my mood lightening slightly, and then at one point Phyllis smiled. Suddenly—

as if the mood angel were watching over me, deciding that I'd brooded quite long enough—I realized that Phyllis was gorgeous.

Not handsome. Not attractive. Not pretty.

Drop-dead gorgeous.

Then I further realized who she was.

Miss America.

When da Vinci devised his theory of facial balance and perfection (the face dividing equally into forehead, middle third, and lower third), he could easily have had Phyllis George in mind. The shape of her eyes slanted up, slightly. Her upper eyelids had a little fullness, which I could tell was natural, something she'd always had. Unlike the typical fifty-year-old, she had no bags under her eyes. Her bone structure was incredible. She had great skin, with her trademark dimples. Her jawline was smooth.

Later, she would tell me she was taken aback by me, unfamiliar as she was with the phenomenon of a man ignoring her.

I perked up, as if out of a months-long stupor.

"This is very bizarre," I told her, "but we met once before, ten years ago, in this very restaurant, Demarchelier, only when it was downtown."

She looked at me foggily.

"We had the same real estate broker," I continued with renewed energy now, "and we looked at the same apartment that day. I never forgot you." I'm sure she thought I was making it up, since I had pretty much ignored her from the start of the evening. "I can tell you the length of your hair that day ten years ago, the dress you wore, the color of your lipstick, everything about you from the first moment I saw you."

She looked at me. "If there ever was a line to knock a girl over," she said, "man, you delivered it." But I could tell she still didn't quite buy it.

"You wore a blue sequined top," I said. "A black skirt. Pearl earrings. Pearl necklace. Your hair was shoulder length. Your lipstick was deep red."

Phyllis looked at me, speechless and blushing.

After dinner I walked Phyllis and Pat outside. I had to go back to the office. They got in a cab. Just before it drove away, Phyllis rolled down her window.

"What's your name again?" she asked.

In a Zone

▼ ▼ ▼

My office was really humming again. Tuesdays and Fridays, as always, were my major surgery days (face-lifts, implants, more extensive lipos). Wednesday mornings I would do small procedures: little biopsies, moles, smaller lipos, fat grafts, and wrinkle removal with collagen, Restylane, Botox, and fat. My other office hours were spent preparing for surgeries—going over photographs, making notes, creating a plan. When I wasn't operating or preparing for surgery, I met with consults and involved myself in the nonsurgical end of the practice.

I was lucky to have such a proficient staff. Giselle, my OR nurse, was responsible for preparing the operating room for the procedures, cleaning the surgical instruments, and wheeling the patients into the OR (I always prepped them for surgery). Lisa or Bob, my treasured anesthesiologists, were in charge of anesthesia and light sedation, and maintaining the crash cart, which included a defibrillator. To date, we have never had to use it, but it is always checked and ready to go. Stella and four other private-duty nurses were called on to help patients recover from major surgery (facelift, breast reduction, abdominal surgery, multiple procedures) by staying with them for at least twenty-four hours postprocedure. For those who don't care about cost, the nurses may stay longer. The nurses monitor the patient's vital signs, check bleeding, hold ice packs, and adjust dressings.

Tanya, my office manager in the Park Avenue office, and Denise, up in Westchester, handled all initial inquiries from prospective patients. Many of them had questions about my background, experience, where I'd graduated from, what my specialties were, etc. For patients already scheduled, one of the office managers would call them about a week before their operation to give instructions (for instance, no aspirin or vitamin E within seven days of the operation, because it promotes bleeding; no food or drink within eight hours before surgery; keep taking any heart medicines, stop taking certain antidepressives; etc.) and to tell them what to bring on the day of their procedure (loose clothing, hat or scarf, sunglasses). The patient was reminded to have someone to pick her up afterward. If the patients were especially nervous, I would speak to them. It's the doctor's job to calm pre-op fears and allay worries about problems that could develop. Patients usually wanted to speak only with me if they had intimate questions they'd been too embarrassed to ask (e.g., When can we start having sex again, and what positions are forbidden for now? Is it okay to take Viagra within days of a face-lift?).

I continued my work as an attending surgeon at Manhattan Eye, Ear & Throat Hospital. I was teaching a course at Cornell, in nerve anatomy.

This was how I liked it. Busy.

Phyllis George and I became friends (not romantically). We often dined together, and I enjoyed her company immensely. Across my twenty years in private practice, I'd developed a special weakness for women from Texas—Houston, Dallas, Fort Worth, San Antonio, Lubbock, Laredo. Each of them was elegant, genial, attractive, smart, sensationally feminine; at least, those in my practice are. It was no surprise to me that Phyllis was from Denton, Texas.

Phyllis invited me to the Kentucky Derby, which she'd told me so much about. Since she'd once been Kentucky's first lady, married to then-governor John Y. Brown, I couldn't think of a better person to experience the event with.

We flew out of New York on a private jet, and other friends of hers joined us. On the tarmac, I fell immediately into conversation with an Austrian gentleman named Helmut, who, it turned out, was married to Susan Lucci, the longtime star of *All My Children*. As his beautifully put-together soap-star wife approached in a gorgeous hat, I called out, *"Guten morgen, Frau Lucci!"* She was taken aback by the greeting, but Helmut beamed. Then Phyllis and Ivana Trump approached, both also in spectacular hats and dressed to kill—Phyllis in a light blue Escada suit, Ivana in a light gray Chanel with a broad collar.

Ivana was immediately likable—funny, smart, great legs. It wasn't long before our conversation turned to her ex-husband, then to marriage. "You know, I really don't need to marry again," said Ivana. "All I need is a cute guy."

After landing in Louisville, we loaded into a stretch limo to Churchill Downs. At the racetrack, the chauffeur came around to open the door, and suddenly it was no longer a day at the races but a crush of humanity. Hundreds, even thousands, of people were milling about the entrance we'd pulled up to. Almost all of them were men, boisterous, ready for a good time. Ivana was the first one to step out of the limo. She pulled teasingly at her skirt, crossed her great legs—posing for a moment so they could bask in the sight—said, "Boys, I'm here!" and stepped out of the limo. You couldn't count the whistles and catcalls. Not to be outdone, Susan Lucci stepped out of the car and exclaimed, as only a seasoned performer could, "Don't forget about me!" then catwalked down what had turned into a makeshift runway through the crowd. Now, with the fans in a frenzy, Phyllis—Miss America, Kentucky's former first lady—emerged and blew off the roof.

I understood what it must have been like for Moses when the Red Sea parted. I was invisible but happy to follow in the wake of these three gorgeous women, who marched up to the VIP lounge, where former Kentucky governor John Brown—Phyllis's ex-husband—greeted us all with "These are my people! These are my people!" The lounge was filled with celebrities, but the one I enjoyed most was my future mayor, Michael Bloomberg, who surprised and delighted me by revealing a funny side most New Yorkers don't see, telling several dirty jokes I won't repeat here.

Every day should bring new lessons. The lessons might be sublime or trivial, but you should go to bed feeling as if you've learned something. For example, one week brought these interesting (to me), sometimes useful, certainly random lessons:

Lesson: I am discovering the difference between wealthy women who work and wealthy women who don't. The former tend to follow your instructions; the latter tend not to listen closely. The former realize that swelling during recovery is normal; the latter tend to obsess on trivial details of the recovery. Should a delay or minor problem arise, the former are satisfied by a reasonable explanation; with the latter, no explanation can satisfy.

Lesson: I figured out one reason why plastic surgeons move so well among the successful and powerful. It's not just because we provide a skill they cherish. It's because we're often just about the only one at these receptions—so overstocked with bankers and lawyers—who is *not* competing with them for their job or place in the pecking order. What we do is too specialized, too weird.

Lesson: Women, especially very successful ones, want their plastic surgeon to be empathetic but not a mushball. Come to think of it, that's what they generally want in a partner, too.

Lesson: Almost no TV anchor I have ever operated on has ever come in for body work. What you can't see behind the desk is apparently of little concern to them.

Lesson: Don't believe everything you read. It's coming out now that many women who read a recent story in a women's magazine—about antiwrinkle injections, so popular in France—are now getting infections. When the story came out, I wondered why the reporter hadn't dug deeper; I knew one of the physicians mentioned in the story had been experiencing complications back then!

Lesson: I am learning more in the nerve anatomy course I teach than the students are. We had thirty-two cadavers out today, each for a member of the class, and we dissected out facial nerves. While I was teaching them, I was not only coming up with a new way to dissect nerves faster, but truly appreciating how varied nerves can be—thickness, number of branches, etc.—from person to person. Fascinating.

It just goes to show: Learning must never stop.

I didn't generally witness cosmetic surgery patients engaged in life-and-death struggles.

Lily was thirty-eight when she came to me to have a childhood scar "revised"—that is, to have its thickness and appearance reduced. It was on her right abdomen, the result of an appendectomy. I cut around the scar, loosening the surrounding skin with a scalpel and scissors, then closed the incision by using different sutures in multiple layers. I then sent the scar to the pathology lab, as I routinely do. (It would come back with a normal reading.)

When Lily came in to have the sutures removed, she was happy with the result. She pointed out a second abdominal scar she also wanted revised. This one was on the left abdomen, from an operation she'd had as an adult, a year before, to remove adrenal cancer. It's common particularly for cancer survivors to want scars reduced. The scar reminds them of the cancer, of fear, of mortality.

During this follow-up visit, Lily spoke to me of unusually intimate things—in this case, childhood operations, an embarrassing scar, cancer. Emotionally, it was as if we'd been through ten or twenty encounters, not two. She opened up. She told me she worked in Manhattan as the office manager of an ad agency. She was single. She looked forward to meeting a guy. She hoped to marry someday. She had a lighthearted, bright way about her, rare in a single New York woman in her late thirties.

When Lily came back for her second revision, she was not lighthearted. Lately she'd been feeling sharp abdominal pain, and she was scheduled to see her gynecologist about it. Given her history, there was extra reason to worry. I tried to be as calming as I could without saying things that weren't true.

While I looked at her in the exam room, she was able to forget some of her anxiety. She complained about the lip of fat creeping over the waist of her jeans.

"Maybe I'll get lipo, too, next time," she said. "What do you think?"

I said I'd be happy to do it.

She'd come to my office for a simple procedure, and the motivating factor had been to make her life better, not keep it from getting worse. For a few moments there, it seemed as if I were simply a confidant, not a doctor; she was not worrying over her long-term health. I felt good. I was moved that she could be transported like that.

When she came back two weeks later for the operation to have the second scar revised, she told me they had discovered a mass in her abdomen. Recurrent adrenal cell carcinoma. We canceled the scar revision.

"I'm one of your doctors and I will help take care of you," I told her, seeing the fright in her eyes. "We go on this journey *together.*"

I didn't know how it would go, of course. The course of disease continually surprises. Cells respond to therapy. Cells don't. I don't know if it's accurate even to call Lily a friend. Yet I knew that her next weeks would be very hard, and that I would be getting closer to this woman whose future had just become filled with storm clouds.

That day, I remember, she wore hip, low-cut jeans, a long Armani blouse, delicate silver-hoop earrings. At one point, she gazed out the window, looking hopeful. She felt less alone, she said. She left the office with a smile.

"I'll call after the oncologist's meeting next week," she said.

Six weeks later, Lily was dead.

I never forget that I'm a physician as well as a plastic surgeon. This thought is nurtured by all the lessons learned from my father, from Dr. Sabiston, from all my mentors. When I first see a patient, I know—and sometimes even say aloud—that we're about to embark on a journey together. For some, it's brief; for others, it's longer. For some, it's filled with joy; for others, it's filled with desperation and even tragedy.

For plastic surgeons who don't do just cosmetic surgery but reconstructive surgery, too, experiencing situations like Lily's differentiates us from those who do cosmetic surgery exclusively (dentists, oral surgeons, etc.). I'm not suggesting that the former group should get extra credit: As I said earlier, I believe it's a myth to think that doing a rhinoplasty or a face-lift, say, is somehow less satisfying and honorable than doing a skin graft. It's all about making patients happier.

But I'm also quite sure that having to deal with situations like Lily's enables us to develop a better rapport with our patients. To be more involved and compassionate, because we, like they, may feel more vulnerable. Plastic surgeons—at least on TV and in the tabloids—don't often get portrayed as having great depths of feeling.

Thoughts of Lily and others like her remain with me forever.

No One to Heal

▼ ▼ ▼

Tuesday, September 11, 2001, 8:00 A.M., a gorgeous, clear blue New York fall morning, I was in my operating room, doing a face-lift on Dorothy, a native of Odessa, Texas, and a friend of former first lady Barbara Bush. The operation was proceeding routinely until sometime after eight, when Tanya entered with the portable phone. Chyresse, an old friend from Grosse Pointe who worked as a manager for American Airlines, had a question for me while she was in rush-hour traffic on the George Washington Bridge. Lisa, my anesthesiologist, took the portable and held it to my ear.

I almost never talk on the phone when I'm in the OR, but Chyresse said it was important—a medical emergency concerning one of the flight attendants she supervised. In the middle of her question, she paused and said, "That's very strange . . . one of our planes just flew into restricted airspace. I gotta call ops." And she hung up.

I thought nothing of it.

Twenty minutes later, Tanya came in to tell us that there'd been a report that a plane had hit the World Trade Center. Along with most New Yorkers, for the first moments that morning, I assumed the crash was a terrible accident—though, on such a cloudless day, it was hard to believe.

Maybe ten minutes later Tanya entered the OR again to tell us that a second plane had crashed into the other tower.

"No way that's chance," said Lisa as I continued operating at normal cadence.

Twenty minutes later, Tanya reentered. "One of the towers collapsed," she said, shaken.

For the first time all morning, I paused. I looked at Lisa. Her mouth was hidden behind her surgical mask, but her eyes were wide, animated. I returned to Dorothy's face—immobile, serene.

"What about the power supply?" Lisa asked. "Or other attacks?"

I reassured her that we had backup generators and supplies, and that we were in a safe building.

Ten minutes later, Tanya entered the OR with an update that the second tower had collapsed.

"All those people," said Lisa. "All those people . . ." She began to cry.

In my mind I estimated that, if we were very, *very* lucky, there would be only twenty-five thousand dead. Injured in the tens of thousands.

And who knew what other terrorist acts still awaited? There would be a great need for help, particularly medical, and I'd had experience working with burn patients during my residency at New York Hospital and Stanford. I told Tanya to cancel our next two surgeries. I finished Dorothy's face-lift, applied her dressings, and moved her to recovery. For a moment I wondered about her reaction to the news when she awoke.

Everything's fine, Dorothy, you were great, face looks fabulous, bruising minimal, twenty thousand dead, the World Trade Center is no more, America is under siege. And remember: ice packs for the first twenty-four hours.

I wondered just how close she was to the Bushes.

Tanya and I checked our office supply of flashlights and batteries, and I gave her money to go buy water and food in case they sealed the city and we were all trapped at the office; my staff lived in

Staten Island, Queens, and Connecticut. A news report instructed all doctors to report to their affiliated or nearby hospitals. I told everyone to stay in the office.

Outside it was dreamlike. The feeling was nothing like I imagined it must be downtown, but still it was eerie. No cars moving on Park Avenue, no taxis hurtling to make it through a just-turned red light. For the first time since I'd opened my office on Park and Sixty-fifth a decade ago, I absorbed the significance of the building just two blocks up the wide boulevard from me: the Sixty-seventh Street Armory. The police had sealed off streets. The National Guard was out on Park Avenue, with M16s at their hips. I needed to get to St. Vincent's Hospital, the hospital closest to the crash site. I explained to a policeman that I had to get downtown. He didn't even ask for ID. He asked permission from his superior officer, who immediately granted it, and we jumped into a cruiser and drove at breakneck speed down the empty avenue. Thousands of people streamed uptown on foot.

At Thirteenth Street, people were jammed outside St. Vincent's Hospital, waiting in front of placards that read *A+, A−, B, B−, O,* donating blood. Everyone was obedient, silent. They must have come from all over the city.

"Good luck, Doc," said the policeman as I hopped out. As if by instinct, we both simultaneously saluted each other.

Given the volume of people milling about, it was disturbingly quiet; inside the Grosse Pointe Central Library on a lazy summer afternoon, with the windows open, might have been louder. Every honking car had gone quiet, every know-it-all New Yorker had become a foot soldier straining to be told where to go to help.

The silence was broken by two jet fighters coming in low, each with full missile payloads. They were the first wave—Air Guard. Then came the U.S. Air Force, a fuller squadron of fighters in formation, all loaded with live air-to-air missiles.

It was eleven thirty in the morning.

Sadly, I stood around for hours with nothing to do, no one to help. As did all the doctors and nurses there. No one was brought into the ER. We all just waited outside for survivors who never came. We knew there had been mass casualties; we didn't know they had already been vaporized. Or that the number of hurt (or dead) not in the buildings was shockingly low. Now and then, in a scattered funereal march, dazed policemen and firemen would tramp by, covered with soot; every now and then a bystander would run over to them to offer a towel or a handkerchief to wipe them off.

After standing there for three hours and realizing that no one was coming, I began the walk uptown. People on the street were crying. They crowded into bars, staring at TVs tuned to the news. At the Fifty-ninth Street Bridge there was a mass of humanity, thousands of people crossing over. On Madison and Sixty-fourth, I barely recognized an Andover classmate covered in soot. He was an investment banker who worked at Deutsche Bank downtown and had been a great runner in school. Dazed, he told me he had just stepped out the front door of his office building as the first tower crumbled before his eyes. Then he ran the fastest mile of his life.

On Fifth Avenue, there were still no cars, and I experienced something for the first time in my almost two decades of living and working in New York City, something I did not even know I was missing all these years.

I heard birds singing in Central Park.

Later, after I checked on the office and saw that everyone was okay, and as the clear blue sky turned golden on that ghastly day, and the acrid stench turned north, and the reality of it began to creep in, I headed downtown once more. I got turned away at Canal Street. Construction trucks were lined all the way back up the tip of Manhattan, a fusillade of Good Samaritans: national guardsmen, construction workers, ironworkers.

Meanwhile, at practically all of the city's population hubs—the Empire State Building, Penn Station, Port Authority, etc.—one bomb threat after another kept setting off building evacuations. A bomb threat at Grand Central Station was called in. The adjoining buildings, including the Grand Hyatt just above the station, were evacuated. Dorothy, who that beautiful morning so long ago had had her face lifted, who had slept through probably the single most traumatizing, deadly day in the history of America, who was healing with bandages on her face in a hotel suite on the forty-fourth floor, was escorted down the elevator by Giselle, my nighttime nurse assigned to her. In the further surreality in front of the Grand Hyatt, standing there all bandaged up, a young policeman approached Dorothy, probably assuming she'd been injured in the chaos of the day.

"Ma'am, do you need a doctor?" he asked.

Dorothy shook her head, wrapped in an Ace-like bandage.

"What a day," he said.

She nodded. "I missed most of it," she said quietly.

"Lucky you," said the cop.

The Limitations
of Plastic Surgery
▼ ▼ ▼

The young, beautiful wife of a director of one of L.A.'s most prominent museums came to me, wanting her near-perfect breasts lifted and slightly reduced.

"Don't," I told her. "Leave them. It won't improve them very much at all. You'll be left with scars. The improvement is not worth it. Please reconsider."

She went to a colleague of mine, who did it.

A year later, she came back to me. Her breasts were flatter. She had wide scars. Her nipples were numb.

"Fix them," she begged, verging on tears.

I could improve but not eradicate the scars, I told her, and I could partially correct the volume loss of her breasts. I could not restore the sensation to her nipples.

She was beside herself.

From the outset, you know some patients will never be happy. Others, you can't tell. Only afterward do you find out how unrealistic they were about what plastic surgery was going to do for them.

You didn't pull me enough. You didn't take out enough fat.

One man with a 34 waist came in for lipo. Then he sued me because he felt uncomfortable in size 32 pants, even though I had never promised he would go down a pants size. (The case was thrown out.)

Sometimes, postoperative denial sets in. Jason's nose had deviated more than an inch to the left. That's not a misprint—*an inch*—having been broken several times from basketball injuries and biking. I corrected it significantly. After the surgery, it deviated to the left four millimeters. It was as aligned and symmetrical as I could get it. Any more wasn't possible because the scar tissue and the thickness of the cartilage limited what I could do.

"You can do better," Jason insisted.

"Actually, I can't," I told him. "It's the best I can do."

Despite the major improvement, Jason was unhappy—angry actually. I showed him his pre-op photos so he could see how far we'd come.

He looked at the photos. He shook his head. "That's not me."

"Yes, it is," I said.

"No," said Jason. "It's not."

It was.

I need to do touch-ups on about 5 percent of my surgeries. It happens most frequently with liposuction because you simply can't feel every nuance of fat. Or the patient may come back because of a scar she doesn't like, or there's a slight bump left on the nose. Touch-ups don't happen often, they're never major, and they're done under local anesthesia.

One of my pet peeves is doing a touch-up after lipo—not because I don't want to do it but because the patient may come to me under false pretenses.

When Nina came in initially for liposuction, she weighed 116 pounds. I lipoed three pounds off her abdomen and hips.

Three months later, she returned, complaining that the lipo hadn't worked. She demanded a redo.

I put her on the scale. She now weighed 126.5 pounds. If in the weeks after lipo she'd come in heavier than her pre-lipo weight, that would have been normal, the result of swelling. But this was three months later.

I asked Nina a number of questions, finally eliciting that she'd been drinking lots of protein shakes and beer. I promised I'd do a free touch-up for her if she lost weight and got down to her pre-lipo 116.

She never returned. Not infrequently, people think that liposuction is a license to eat badly and not exercise. These people are just kidding themselves. Lipo will never work for them because the fat will always find new places to deposit.

Two weeks after doing a face-lift on Gabrielle, a somewhat homely woman in her early forties, I got a call from her mother, who was extremely upset.

"She doesn't look like my daughter anymore," she complained.

It would be a serious complaint if it were true.

I talked calmly to the mother, but she was furious and wouldn't listen. "No!" she said angrily. "The point isn't whether Gabrielle looks good or not. It's that she no longer looks like my daughter!"

I'd been particularly happy with the outcome of that lift; as usual, I'd gone for the natural, subtle improvement, not a dramatic change. Afterward, I thought Gabrielle looked terrific. So did my staff.

But her mother was not assuaged.

She continued to call the office for a week, ranting at me for taking away her daughter. (I did not hear from Gabrielle herself.) She threatened to sue me.

Mother and daughter went to see a lawyer, armed with before-and-after pictures. The lawyer wouldn't take the case; he said Gabrielle looked great in the afters, and they had no case.

I knew this because the lawyer called me the next day.

"Can I bring in my girlfriend?" he asked.

I did not hear from Gabrielle's mother again.

Sometimes, there is simply nothing that anyone can do.

Not plastic surgery. Not the exercising of willpower. Not the best of intentions.

If love doesn't want to flourish, I discovered, it simply won't.

So what do you do then? If you're a person who loves life, you look for someone else to love.

I watched it happen.

Jeanette Longoria, my patient many times over (face-lift, eye lift, abdominal liposuction) and now a good friend, is a vivacious woman in her seventies. After she'd been widowed for some time, she became eager for male companionship, and met a retired ambassador from the United Nations. She was crazy about him. He was handsome, charming, learned, interesting, spoke nine languages—and he was crazy about her. He asked her to dinner. When he picked her up at her apartment, he was armed with a huge bouquet of yellow roses. While drinking champagne over dinner, he leaned over and kissed her. She smiled at him.

He called again the next night. *Could he take her out to dinner?* he wanted to know. This time the roses were pink. On the walk home after dinner, the retired ambassador once again bent to kiss her. She felt cold shivers up and down her arm.

She told me about it on the phone the next day. "What happened?" she asked. I thought I knew but I didn't say. The retired ambassador had asked Jeanette to dinner again that night. She would report to me what happened.

Red roses this time. Jeanette and the ambassador went to a show, then dinner, and again he kissed her. The hair on her arm stood up.

I saw her the next afternoon. "I don't know what to do," she said to me. "He's everything I love in a man. *More*. What's going on?"

"It's pheromones," I told her, and she reluctantly nodded, as if she had already figured it out, too. It had happened to me, once. I went out with a lawyer—smart, interesting, pretty, everything—and each time I leaned over to kiss her . . . nothing.

"You might as well quit now," I told her. "No matter what you do, it won't change."

She shook her head. She knew I was right.

So what did she do about it?

At seventy years old, she wrote a book about finding romance and sensuality at any age. She's inspired not only her family and friends, but widows, divorcées, and older women around the country, who now flock by the hundreds to her book readings and signings.

Maybe there always *is* something you can do, after all, so long as you've got the attitude.

The Politician and the First Lady

▼ ▼ ▼

Politicians and royalty—more than movie stars or the very wealthy—are the most secretive people I work with.

I was contacted by the friend of one of America's most influential and high-profile elected officials. Not by a staff member; it's never a staff member. They're not trusted with real secrets. The politician's friend and I, on my cell phone, worked out all the details for the meeting.

When the elected official came to my office, he showed me what he thought was a melanoma on his shoulder. It looked quite suspicious to me. He was desperately afraid that if word got out, constituents would think he was dying, and it would cost him his upcoming bid for reelection. I did a wider removal than normal and told him I'd send the melanoma off to be biopsied.

"No, you can't do that," he said. "It's not so simple."

"What do you mean?"

"Well, it's going to a lab, correct?"

"Yes."

"People at labs can read. They can see whose name is on it, correct?"

"You don't want this sample attached to you."

"That's correct."

I nodded. "Would you like me to use my name?"

"Correct. And your Social Security number, of course."

"Of course," I agreed.

I sent the mole to the lab, using my Social Security number and name, pretending the sample was my tissue.

It turned out to be a melanoma "in situ"—a mole with some changes—but the wider removal did the trick. The paranoid politician was in the clear.

In November of 2002, he would win re-election.

Deirdre, an investment banker, age thirty-five, came in for breast augmentation.

"I want the biggest implants you can put in that still allows the skin to close around it," she said.

She was a borderline case. I considered turning her away, something I do to maybe one in seven people who walk through the door for a consultation, when I don't see the problem they do or significantly disagree with the result they're going for.

But Deirdre had a wide pelvis and narrow shoulders, and her frame could handle what she was asking for. Structurally and aesthetically it was what she wanted, not to mention what her boyfriend wanted. She was resolute. When patients are unequivocal about what they want, I've found, the outcome is usually happy.

Several months later, Deirdre returned to my office, unhappy.

"I want them *bigger,*" said Deirdre, though it looked as if she had two medicine balls on her chest.

"I won't do it," I told her.

She tried to persuade me but I stood my ground. She called a few days later to report, almost petulantly, that she'd found someone near Gramercy Park who was willing to give her bigger implants. Finding a surgeon willing to perform virtually any procedure is not something to be proud of, I wanted to tell her, for patient *or* doctor.

Deirdre was not a risk I wanted to take.

▼

In October of 2002, my friend Janet Carlson called from Los Angeles. "Nancy Reagan would like to meet you for lunch," she informed me.

"Any time that pleases Mrs. Reagan would be fine for me," I said. I held the first lady in high esteem.

While crossing the country, I worried about our conversation. I like to try to put people at ease and I was interested in meeting her. But what would I say? Everything had been said. It was an incredibly difficult stage in Mrs. Reagan's life. Obviously she was suffering terribly as she watched her beloved husband endure the advanced stages of Alzheimer's disease. Whatever anyone may have thought of his or her politics, theirs was one of the great American romances of the last half century. I'd read his book of love letters to her and found them inspiring.

What subject could I bring up to interest her? Her work for a drug-free America? Her growing interest in stem-cell research? The upcoming midterm elections?

Somewhere over Kansas I remembered that her stepfather, Loyal Davis, had been a brilliant neurosurgeon, chairman of the surgery department at Northwestern University, and president, for years, of the American College of Surgeons. When I'd trained at Duke, there was a Loyal Davis Ward. That was my icebreaker.

When I got to L.A., I picked up my pal Janet and we proceeded to Spago, the famous Wolfgang Puck restaurant on Sunset Boulevard. Mrs. Reagan sat at a table in the far corner surrounded, at a casual distance, by Secret Service agents. From the front of the restaurant she looked tiny and frail.

Janet and I walked over and she introduced us. The first lady *was* tiny and frail, but smartly dressed in a red tweed suit. She showed physical signs of aging, of course, but she was still beautiful—good bone structure and a twinkle in her eyes; her personality shined through. She was sharp and intelligent and had a singular poise. She emanated a quietness to her physical being, and a worldliness. On that day, more than anything, Mrs. Reagan appeared sad. Almost as soon as we'd exchanged pleasantries, her daughter, Patti, an attractive brunette, fifty, swooped into the restaurant and sat down with the three of us. You could see right away how fun she was, but her electricity, especially in that setting, threw me off guard. When something unexpected happens in the OR, I am always prepared; for the unexpected in life, I'm not nearly so adaptable.

"I was a problem child," said Patti, natural as can be. We'd hardly gotten past *Hello my name is Patti Hi I'm Cap* when she offered the frank self-analysis. I was fascinated by her. "Just before my father was inaugurated governor of California," she said, "I ran off with the drummer for the Eagles. Just before my father was inaugurated president, I did a spread in *Playboy*." She paused for only the briefest moment; it was touching, almost funny, how public her disturbances had been, and impressive how aware of it she was.

"And now," said Patti with a smile, "I'm happy to take care of my dad and to be with my mother."

It was a moment of almost unbearable feeling—at that table, at that moment, there was so much love and regret, acceptance and maturity, intimacy and reflection. More than anything, though, I could feel the sadness that mother and daughter were both experiencing about their respective husband and father, a foreboding.

I felt it was time, so I asked Mrs. Reagan about her stepfather the surgeon. Her eyes lit up. She launched into a series of stories about her dad's days at Northwestern, and what it was like when he came home after a long day at the hospital. The somber mood at our table had broken, if only for a while, and we started to have a good time. I thought of how basic a bond Mrs. Reagan and I shared— both having grown up in the Midwest with hardworking doctors for fathers, fathers whose devotion to their patients and profession meant they often didn't have time for their family.

A friend of mine—a noted screenwriter and also a patient—entered the restaurant and spotted me, walked toward the table . . . and his eyebrow raised at the ominous federal agents surrounding my lunch partners and me. He then recognized the first lady, introduced himself, and did me a big favor. "Mrs. Reagan, this guy here is the only honest plastic surgeon in town," he said. As soon as he left, another friend—heiress to a great retail fortune—also walked in and noticed me, and she, too, came over. She also knew Mrs. Reagan, it turned out.

"Nancy, this is the man I was telling you about," she said, then turned to me. "Please hold me a spot."

She smiled and left.

You can't buy advertising like this, I thought. One of the Secret Service agents eyed me suspiciously. I wondered if he thought I'd planted friends to appear at appropriate intervals and say nice things.

Mrs. Reagan looked at me wistfully. "Oh, plastic surgery. I would love to do something, you know. God knows I could use it. But I could never have it while my husband's sick. Can you imagine if I had any work done—and he died?" Now she focused on me forcefully. "He demands my full attention. I just can't."

After two hours of nostalgia and lunch and a chance to forget the trouble that awaited her back home in Santa Barbara, Mrs. Reagan, along with her daughter, said so long to Janet and me and parted, their Secret Service detail in tow.

That night, I returned to New York on the overnight. I drifted off to sleep thinking of Mrs. Reagan and what might happen to her.

▼

Several months later, I was doing late-afternoon paperwork in my office when Tanya buzzed me. A call from the New York City Police Department, a Detective Amarosa. I picked up.

"Dr. Lesesne, is Deirdre MacNeil your patient?" he asked.

"Yes."

"When did you last operate on her?"

"About eight months ago."

"Can you tell me her breast implant serial number?"

My stomach dropped. Why was he asking about her breast implants? How did he know she had breast implants?

"Breast implants don't have serial numbers on them," I replied. "Only the size in cc's printed on the bottom of the implants."

Pretty much anything that came out of his mouth next, I braced myself, would be bad.

"Why?" I asked.

"We believe she went to an unlicensed surgeon for work, the operation went awry and she died, and the surgeon panicked, cut her into pieces, and put her in a suitcase, which we found buried under the surgeon's garage in New Jersey."

We're All Alike

▼ ▼ ▼

I was invited to a wedding in Turkey. My friend Cemile's daughter was getting married. I had done a face-lift on Cemile back when she was married; she'd since gotten divorced. It was a Muslim wedding, a chic and elegant crowd, with guests from every part of Turkish society. The sun was setting over the Sea of Marmara, illuminating the Dolmabahce Palace. The ceremony was incredibly short—maybe two minutes in all—with the mayor of Istanbul presiding. After he pronounced the couple husband and wife, a flock of doves was released over the Bosphorus.

Dinner and dancing would last until morning. There were devout Muslims there who didn't drink, though they were dressed in Western fashion. Across the grand room, I spotted the sister of a woman I'd done a breast augmentation on three years before. But after the woman's husband had become a fundamentalist, he'd insisted she have the implants removed. She came to my office. At first I resisted: The implants were perfect—soft and natural-looking. But the woman demanded, and nothing I was going to say would dissuade her. Forlornly, I took them out—the only time in twenty years that, short of a medical concern, I've removed implants.

The wedding reception that Cemile and her ex-husband were throwing for their daughter was more elegant than opening night at the Metropolitan Opera. What a gorgeous moment this was, especially for Cemile.

Or should have been.

In her yellow Givenchy dress, Cemile came over to me. "Would you dance with me?" she asked. I said of course. Cemile's eyes were grateful as I led her out onto the dance floor.

When we were out there, Cemile moved her mouth close to my ear. "My ex-husband is here with his young girl," she whispered. I looked at her. She smiled.

I danced with her all night long.

We really are all alike.

Sure, I deal often with the superrich and the famous and the fabulous, with patients whose very livelihoods depend on looking gorgeous and youthful. The universe they inhabit operates, in many ways, almost nothing at all like the one inhabited by the vast majority of the world. But—as I said earlier—everybody's got something. I do, you do, they do, we all do. Something that annoys, something that disheartens. That commonality cuts across wealth, status, ability. And the reasons my patients seek cosmetic surgery are (with the occasional odd exception) few and fundamental. To buy time. To recapture youth. To banish insecurity. To prolong a career. To stave off depression. To gain entry to new experiences, new business, new relationships. When they call me, when they're sitting across from me in my office, when they're lying beneath me on the table in my OR, it's because there's *something* that's driven them to distraction. The very rich and the not rich, the average-looking and the drop-dead gorgeous.

We're all alike.

Now and then, at the end of an especially long day, a day when I've been up at five in the morning, completed three face-lifts and find myself at the office past nine doing paperwork, an image of my father, Dr. John Lesesne, the family internist, comes to me. He is in his office working late, just like me, doctor to doctor. His dedication—the quality that kept him from me so often growing up that I resisted pursuing medicine until I couldn't any longer . . . his dedication has become my dedication. By the time he was my age, he had a big family, and I do not. But his love of medicine is now mine. His intense work ethic is now mine. His single-minded devotion to patients is now mine.

I hoped that I could catch lightning in a bottle. After dating a lovely woman for two years, I decided I was ready again to try marriage.

I proposed.

The World Is My Museum
▼ ▼ ▼

Autumn.

The best New York season, end of discussion. It's a particularly crisp fall day, with the faint smell of woodsmoke in the air. Yellow, orange, and red leaves are scattered like handprints across Fifth Avenue. A perfect day for a crunchy Michigan Red Delicious apple, or a New York McIntosh.

I have just come from the Metropolitan Museum of Art, where I'd popped in for forty-five soothing, invigorating minutes studying and luxuriating in the beautiful paintings, particularly the portraits.

I walk briskly to my office. With so little free time, walking to and from the office is one of my stolen pleasures, doubling as exercise and head-clearing.

Do you really have time for me?

That's what she had said in response to my marriage proposal. I knew it was really just a polite way of saying no.

After many years of being single-minded (figuratively and literally), I had thought I was ready to embark on a new personal journey—marriage and family. Unfortunately, the woman I'd hoped would join me on the journey was not in the same frame of mind. Timing is everything.

Another lesson learned.

Yet my soul was nourished, continually so. I thought of Dr. Henry Ransom, the accomplished professor emeritus of surgery at the University of Michigan who'd given me, at age nineteen, a chance to work in his department, the first step in the series of steps that had led to my fulfilling my professional and creative dream. When I'd met Dr. Ransom in his eighties—white-haired, distinguished—he had already lived a wonderful, productive life. He had been a great general surgeon and an excellent teacher. He had touched the lives of many surgeons and doctors and patients, who had in turn touched many more. As to that little matter of his not having found time to have a family himself? So what?

My father had. Dr. Ransom had not. Dr. Sabiston had.

Hard-driving doctors all. Good lives all.

The deepest unifying theme for the three of them, I thought, was this: They'd all led lives of dedication.

It is late afternoon and the light is turning golden. The reflections off the high windows soften, and shadows slant across people's faces. I walk a block east, to Madison, and now stroll down the west side of the avenue, passing the elegant antiques stores of the high Seventies. The sidewalks are not so crowded that it's one big mass of people. Instead, you can see them individually. It's a touch wintry outside and people are bundled up. It's not easy to get a sense of their bodies.

I concentrate, as always, on their faces.

I try first to make them out from far away. From a distance, the first thing I notice is the overall shape of the face.

Her's is an almost perfect oval.

He's got a square jawline.

Her neck is too soft.

The next thing I notice, as they get closer, is the animation.

His eyebrows arch unusually high.

Her lips pucker asymmetrically.

As they get closer still, I notice the size of the lips.

Then the eyes.

Then the textures. Of skin. Scars. Hair.

I scan passing New Yorkers as if they are each a painting in a museum, but paintings that change from instant to instant—

nuanced changes in their movement, their expression, the failing sunlight, my own perception.

She's one of those beautiful ones with almost preternaturally clear eyes. And though her chin is small, it's not weak.

He's got a Latin complexion but the jaw anatomy of an Eastern European.

Wow, she looks angry. If I could only do an endo browlift on her, she'd stop scaring her friends and coworkers.

Just before they pass, gone forever, I discreetly glance sideways, for one last, different angle.

What a nasal hump.

Uneven pigmentation.

A slight—and sexy—overbite.

I can't help myself. This is who I am.